EXTREME
TRAINING

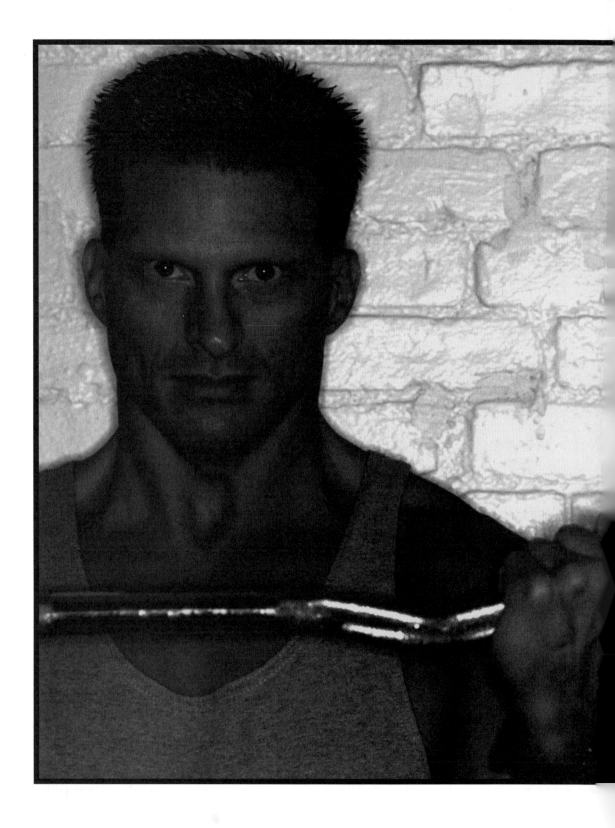

BRAD HAMLER'S
EXTREME TRAINING

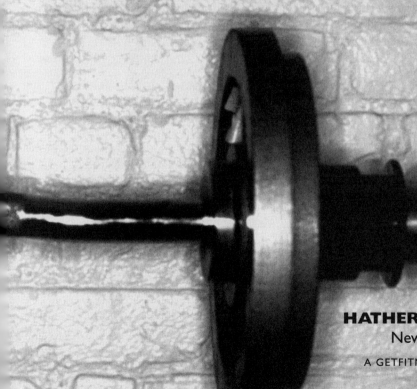

HATHERLEIGH PRESS
New York, NY
A GETFITNOW.COM BOOK

Extreme Training: Taking Fitness to the Max

A GETFITNOW.COM BOOK

Hatherleigh Press/Getfitnow.com Books
An Affiliate of W.W. Norton & Company, Inc.
5-22 46th Ave. Suite 200
Long Island City, NY 11101
1-800-528-2550

Visit our website:
www.getfitnow.com

> **DISCLAIMER:** Before beginning any exercise program consult your physician. The author and publisher of this book and workout disclaim any liability, personal or professional, resulting from the misapplication of any of the training procedures described in this publication.

All Getfitnow.com titles are available for bulk purchase, special promotions, and premiums. For more information, please contact the manager of our Special Sales Department at 1-800-528-2550.

Library of Congress Cataloging-in-Publication Data

Hamler, Brad.
    Extreme training / Brad Hamler.
      p. cm.
    ISBN 1-57826-062-0 (alk. paper)
    1. Physical fitness—Handbooks, manuals, etc. 2. Exercise—Handbooks, manuals, etc.
    3. Physical education and training—Handbooks, manuals, etc. I. Title.
    GV481 .H24 2001
    613.7'1—dc21
                                                2001016784
                                                    CIP

Cover design by Peter Gunther
Text design and composition by John Reinhardt Book Design
Photography by Peter Field Peck with Canon® cameras and lenses
on Fuji® print and slide film

Printed on acid-free paper

10 9 8 7 6 5 4 3 2 1

Printed in Canada

To all the clients I've trained over my 18-year career, whose hard work, inspiration, and support made this book possible.

And to Katja, the best kid in the world.

ACKNOWLEDGMENTS

First and foremost, I thank my publisher, Hatherleigh Press, for giving me the opportunity to bring *Extreme Training*—my story and philosophy—to light. This project also would not have been possible without the extraordinary contributions of my editor, Heather Ogilvie. Her abilities to interpret the mass of information I threw at her and to organize my thoughts as they flew at breakneck speed were truly amazing.

I'd also like to thank the organization and person responsible for providing me with the basis of my training and biomechanical knowledge: the National Academy of Sports Medicine (NASM) and Tom Purvis, who had a life-altering impact on my ideas about what truly constitutes exercise.

Finally, I'm grateful to both photographer Peter Field Peck for his talent in capturing my ideas about exercise on film and James C. Villepigue for support during the photo shoot and production of *Extreme Training*.

Brad Hamler
February 2001

CONTENTS

From football player to competitive bodybuilder to avid golfer, how I
learned just how far I could push myself—and the right and wrong ways
of doing it.

With so many exercise fads out there today, it's easy to fall prey to
fitness misinformation. Here, we'll discuss the basics of biomechanics
and exercise that will serve as the foundation for lifelong fitness.

The exercise that works tends to be the one that you will do. Here's a
guide to what certain exercises accomplish and how you can arrange
them into an effective, challenging workout that you'll enjoy doing. If
you understand the principles behind creating an exercise program, you
can create a new program whenever you get bored or want more of a
challenge.

These photos and descriptions include outdoor and home-based
exercises to show how the workout fits into an active lifestyle that does
not necessarily have to revolve around the gym.

You're healthy, you're fit, you're able to perform your sport with maximum enjoyment and live your life with gusto. But you still want to challenge yourself. You want to know what separates Olympians and elite athletes from the rest of us. You want to push yourself that last 10 percent of the way to your full physical potential. At this point, your physical future depends on your mental discipline.

x

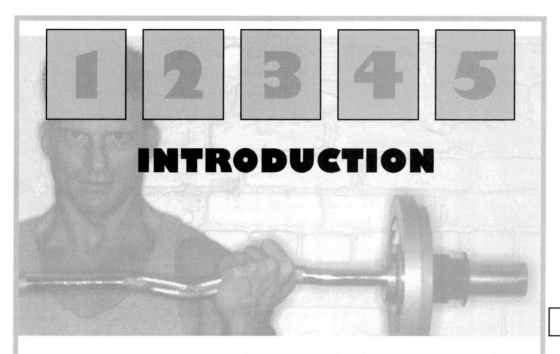

INTRODUCTION

DO YOU WANT TO BE MORE than just a weekend warrior? Have you been exercising for months or years, but after an initial improvement in weight, strength, or endurance, have you seemed to hit a physical "plateau"? Is your workout just not working out anymore? Do you want to go to the next level of fitness—to develop the strength and endurance so that you approach your maximum physical potential?

Whether you want to improve your athletic ability—be it for basketball, mountain biking, tennis, snowboarding, golf, skiing, or extreme sports—or just improve and maximize your overall health and well-being, *Extreme Training* can get you there.

Guys, ever wonder what it's like to have the strength of Mike Piazza? The endurance of Michael Jordan? The versatility of decathlete Dan O'Brien? Ladies, ever wonder what it's like to have the strength of Gabrielle Reese? The endurance of Mia Hamm? The versatility of Jackie Joyner-Kersee? You don't need expensive personal trainers, coaches, exercise gizmos, or eight hours a day to spend in the gym. You just need the will and commitment to maintaining lifetime maximum fitness.

The truth is, a lot of athletes dedicated to their sport fail to complement their training with a regular workout program that includes strength and cardiovascular training. Even regular gym-goers tend to get stuck in a rut,

> The Extreme Training Workout is designed for those who have reached a basic fitness level and can do the following easily:
>
> **MEN**
> Bench press 185 lbs., 8 to 10 reps.
> Do 100 crunches.
> Jog 3.5 miles in 30 minutes.
>
> **WOMEN**
> Bench press 50 lbs.
> Do 100 crunches.
> Jog 3 miles in 30 minutes.

repeating the same exercises and hitting a "wall" they just can't seem to get past. These people are overlooking some basic rules of exercising, and misunderstanding what exercise in general, and what specific exercises in particular, can and cannot do for their bodies.

Extreme Training will get you back to basics, clear up common exercise misconceptions that even seasoned athletes harbor, and help you develop a program that will continue to challenge you.

A lot of people frustrated with their exercise programs try too hard to get over that "wall" or past that "plateau." These folks often end up injuring themselves. *Extreme Training* will show you how to take your fitness to the next level safely and effectively. If an exercise isn't safe, it isn't effective—and chances are, if it's not effective, it's probably not safe.

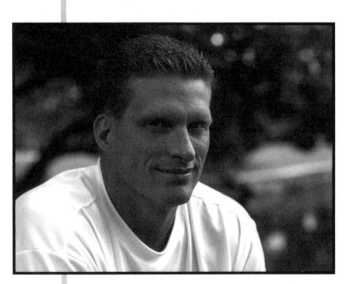

Extreme Training is not about taking yourself to dangerous, unhealthy physical extremes—it's about reaching toward your personal physical potential safely and consistently. To reach that potential safely, you need to understand the "hows" and "whys" of the intended muscle function. That means understanding some basic biomechanics so you'll stop working against your body by "making it" exercise. You'll start working *with* your body to maximize its potential.

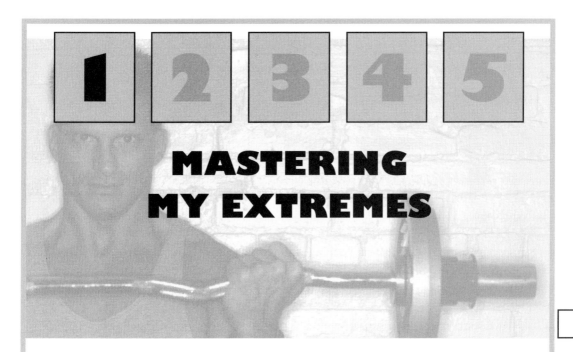

MASTERING
MY EXTREMES

WHEN I WAS EIGHT YEARS OLD, I had an emotionally scarring experience. My mother took me shopping for school clothes, and when we got to

the boys' department at J.C. Penney's, my mom asked the sales lady where a certain size was. The woman looked down at me and said, "Oh, no, this area's not for him. He's a *husky* boy—he needs to go to the husky boys' department."

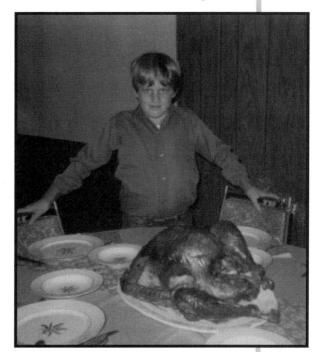

Even to my young ears, the way that she said "husky" seemed to indicate there was something . . . well, *different* about me, and not necessarily in a good way. I didn't want to be known as a "husky boy"; I wanted to be a boy like anybody else. I remember then making the connection between the physiques of athletes (either football players or baseball players) and my physique. "Athletic," I concluded, was the opposite of "husky."

That was when, at age eight, my passion for fitness began.

People get their passion for sports and fitness from different places, and that passion doesn't necessarily start in childhood. Retirees, looking to fill their days and live longer, take up sports and fitness regimes. Baby Boomers, hoping to work off beer bellies and stave off the signs of middle age, hit the gyms. Generation Xers, raised with a heightened awareness of the physical and mental health benefits of exercise, work out on their lunch hours, during their weekends, and even plan physically challenging vacations. Teens and 20-somethings flock to non-traditional "extreme" sports as a way of challenging their physical limits and defining their youth culture. And with a growing population of overweight children, our nation is providing more and more fitness and athletic programs for young kids.

Maybe your passion started with the love for a particular sport. Maybe you were inspired by a famous athlete. Perhaps you took up exercising as a way to lose weight or improve your health. Or maybe you came from an athletic family who encouraged you to participate in sports and maintain your fitness from an early age.

You may not even know when or how exactly you got into fitness. But now you want more. You want more stamina or prowess for your sport, or you want to achieve physical changes that only advanced training can produce. You want to reach your maximum physical potential—with a minimum risk of injury.

Looking back to our childhoods, though, can provide us with clues to our perceptions and "preconceived notions" about exercise. Some of these perceptions can help us build an advanced exercise program that perfectly suits our lifestyles and ambitions. Other perceptions, however, may be false and may perpetuate exercise- and fitness-related myths, ideas that may be holding us back instead of bringing us closer to maximizing our physical potential.

REFLECT ON YOUR ROOTS

I came from a working-class family. Therefore, anything that had to do with working out or pursuing physical activity for its own sake was looked upon as recreation. My father was a carpenter and fireman by trade, and he considered physical sports "extracurricular." He was able to maintain his fitness through the work he did. He was fit, but he wasn't an athlete. In fact, I became the first athlete in my family.

Your grandparents (or perhaps even your parents) probably lived physically demanding lives. If they wanted heat in the winter, they had to go out and cut down a tree for wood. Today, even somebody who's in decent shape, after cutting down a tree and chopping wood, is going to feel it the next day. Believe me, that's exercise!

Our parents and grandparents, therefore, were often too tired from working physically challenging jobs to participate in sports and exercise programs. As a result, many of us didn't see our parents "working out," or even playing sports on their days off. Many of us got our first taste of exercise—for its own sake—from school physical education classes.

In school, football was the first sport that I became serious about. Like many of my classmates, I played basketball in the winter, baseball in the spring, and then football in the fall. By the time I reached the age of eight, having had an epiphany about my "huskiness," I went to my dad and said, "I think it's time that I concentrate on only one sport." And he said, "Well then, you decide what it is you want to do."

Although in the Midwest football is practically a religion, that's not really why I chose it. I truly thought that football was where my potential was; it was what I really enjoyed. My father just stepped back and let me play; he didn't really know anything about sports.

But was school football teaching me about maintaining lifelong fitness? Was it even particularly good at training me for the particular physical rigors of the sport?

At the time, high school coaches and gym teachers didn't really give kids information about exercise. They just said, "This is how to play this sport—now go run out and do it."

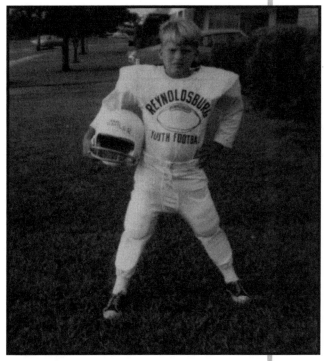

6

That's classic sport-specific training — skills and drills with one sport in mind.

Branded as husky and all, I knew I had to work extra hard to become a good football player. So on my own, I discovered weightlifting. I got my information from what I saw on television. I put my first weight set in my garage—a wobbly little bench and a set of sand-filled plastic weights. In the winter, I'd put on eight sweatshirts, go out in the garage, and lift weights, all on my own.

The poster that came with the weight set had diagrams of the basic weightlifting exercises. Where did *that* information come from? What kind of factual base was a *poster* for someone serious about exercise? I wish I could have one of those posters now so I could look at it and say, "OK, now I know why I am what I am!" The quality of information probably wasn't very good, but at least it pointed me in the right direction. I'm sure lots of other kids, wanting to train for their sport outside of practice and physical education class, turn unsupervised to equipment bought at sporting goods stores and from infomercials, as well as to videos and gyms.

I was even on my own learning to use the multi-purpose Universal machine at my high school. I did manage to get two of my best friends to join me. The three of us had such different body types. I, as you know, was the husky boy; my friend Fran had a wiry, medium-shaped frame; and Doug was scrawny until one day, through the miracle of genetics, he woke up with a tremendous muscular physique and a full beard.

In terms of genes, I probably had the least physical potential of all of us, but I had the strongest work ethic. And through hard work and desire, the tables have turned: I'm working out and maximizing my physical potential; Fran, who's now a chiropractor, is still in pretty decent shape; but Doug, my genetically gifted friend, woke up one day to find himself 30 pounds overweight and bald.

Genetics is, in many ways, destiny. There's not much you can do about the genes that determine your height or your hairline. But with hard work and dedication, you can change your overall physique in terms of your strength and musculature. Likewise, bad habits and laziness can rob you of your genetic potential.

Seeing physical potential in professional athletes was certainly inspirational, but I got a more immediate example of human physical potential—and the wonders of genetics—from a friend's father. This man, Big Bill Miller, was the largest human being I'd ever seen in my life. He was what would now be known as a WWF wrestler. I don't know exactly what his measurements were, but he had to be at least 6'5", over 300 pounds, and a size 22 shoe. He was just a monster of a human being. Having someone that close around gave me the sense that there were physical potentials out there of such extreme. And when you have a mother who's only 4'10" and father who is 5'11", seeing individuals like this obviously challenges your imagination. Back then, I didn't know about genetics, so I just trained harder.

Let's get back to my friends and the high school Universal machine. Being left to our own devices with the machine didn't leave any of us with lifelong injuries, but our lack of training and infor-

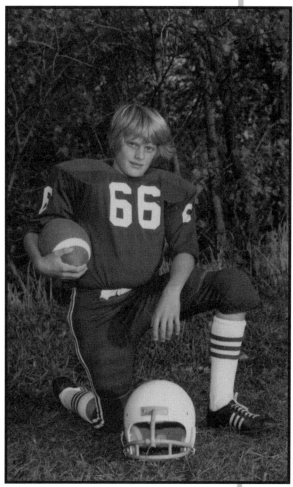

mation easily *could* have led to injury—and certainly slowed us down on our quest for stronger, faster physiques.

My formal education in resistance training started with a gentleman named Steve O'Brien, who owned his own bodybuilding gym. He was the Ohio state champion in power lifting and in bodybuilding. (Today we think of those as two completely different athletes, but at that time bodybuilders and power lifters were the same people. They would bulk up to gain more mass so they could lift heavier weights. Then they'd immediately diet after the power lifting season and begin competitive bodybuilding.) That's where I started getting sensible information about how to approach weight training to specifically build strength for football. (I was not yet training merely for the sake of working out to maximize my potential.)

By my senior year of high school, I lost a lot of my huskiness. I weighed 155 pounds and was 5'11". I had a lot of heart and desire but not the physical attributes of a football player. So I went to Steve to help me "bulk up," so to speak. By the time I entered Findlay College the following fall, I had beefed up to 205 pounds.

That was my first experience in altering my body's composition, and I did it via the old weight-gaining diet and by lifting heavy weights. It was the first time that I felt empowered, that if I really wanted to change my body, I could.

I played back-up linebacker that year, but I was still too small, even at 205 pounds, to be a starting linebacker. The coaches at Findlay said maybe I should play the next year as a defensive back, someone who needs to be smaller and quicker. From my high school years, they remembered me being very quick—so now they wanted me to lose some of the weight I had gained.

Frustrated, I went back to Steve. Here I had spent all that time and energy bulking up! I said, "Steve, now they want me to lose all the weight again — what do I do?" I was lost.

He said, "Oh, that's no big deal. I'll train you like a bodybuilder. I'll get you ripped up."

And that was my first introduction into bodybuilding, where I trained and altered my body composition yet again. I needed to lose the body fat, while maintaining muscle for speed and strength.

This training changed my life, as Steve showed me that there was a whole other sport to training in and of itself. I thought this was great. (This was early 1980s, so I missed out on the heyday of Arnold Schwarzenegger.) I started reading all the books I could get my hands on at that point. But I still hadn't come across any factual, scientific, biomechanical basis for any of the weight-training regimes I did. The books gave sound exercise fundamentals at best, and lucky for me, they worked.

One of the first books that I ever read about training was about Bruce Jenner and how he trained for the decathlon before winning the Gold Medal in the 1976 Olympics and setting a world record. I felt a connection, because I was trying to train for my own sport, all on my own. Jenner had a coach and his wife's support, but he did a lot of his training on his own. So I thought, "OK, there's somebody else out there who's done this already."

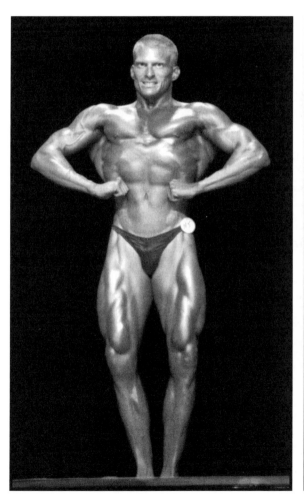
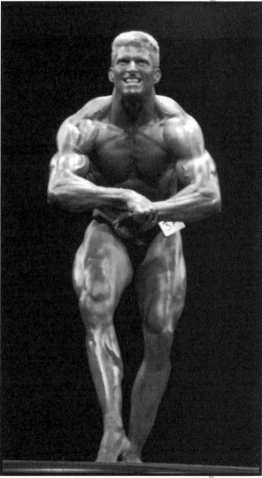

When training didn't work as I'd hoped, I spent many hours by myself questioning why my body was not responding to the training I was putting it through. My sense of frustration that I was not physically fulfilling my potential drove my desire and made me push myself to find those answers.

EXTREME OVERTRAINING

I remember when my hometown got a Nautilus center. The gym guys would go to Nautilus certain days of the week and lift free weights the other days of the week, going back and forth between the two. Looking back in retrospect, I see that we were obviously never letting our bodies recuperate. We were overtraining.

Furthermore, in the summer, I would work 12 hours a day doing a manual labor job—unloading 100 pound bags of sand off trucks for a sandblasting company—then come home, go to the gym, or go to the high school field and run wind sprints or up bleachers. If I had any energy left over, I'd go out and party a little bit.

It was amazing that I could push my body to that extreme and still feel I wasn't really getting anywhere. I still had that feeling of not developing my full physical potential. It's also amazing that I didn't incur any serious injuries. I was very, very lucky.

The first time I did a power lifting squatting-type workout, however, I pushed myself to a physical limitation where I actually became sick. I remember almost passing out in the locker room and then throwing up in the bathroom. I remember thinking to myself that the guys who were training this way were absolute insane animals and that I had to get out of there.

Then Steve and some of the guys came in and said, "Get up off the bathroom floor and go back out to the squat rack immediately!"

And I thought, "You are even more insane than I thought you were—I just threw up! Are you crazy?"

And they said, "If you don't get back out there and do it right now, you never will."

And they were right. They say if you fall off a horse, get right back on, because if you don't you'll never go near another horse for the rest of your life. That was probably the best advice to keep me from abandoning training altogether. But unfortunately, I eventually *got used* to pushing myself to the extent where I would get sick. The idea that you *have* to do that every workout, that you have to push yourself to where you're momentarily physically incapacitated, is not only dangerous, but it's not necessary in order to build toward your physical potential. The phrase "no pain, no gain" is another one of our fitness myths. If you're throwing up, pulling your hamstring, blowing out your knee joint, what exactly do you gain? The only way such activity brings you closer to your physical potential is by *limiting* your potential. The lesson to learn, though, is that when you do go too far, don't abandon the exercise altogether—after rest and rehabilitation, get back out there.

Most people have no concept of what it takes to become sick from physical exertion. Before you'd get to that point, so many impulses would fire in your brain that would tell you to stop, that you would listen and you would stop. It takes tremendous will and drive (and being around psychos who shout, "Keep going! Keep pushing! You can do it!") to find your physical extreme. If you want to reach it bad enough, you will. But do it in a methodical, controlled process—or you may regret it.

QUESTION EVERYTHING

In college, someone once offered me steroids with the advice that steroids would make me bigger, stronger, and faster for football. But I was suspicious. I said, "Well, what else will happen?" I was asking about side effects. Nobody was talking then about damage to the liver, kidney, or heart. But they did say, "Oh, you'll get some acne and your hair will thin out a little bit, and you also may experience some sexual dysfunction."

I said, "That's OK, you can keep the steroids."

A lot of kids today, though, don't hear about even those *non*-life-threatening side effects. And some seem to think bigger muscles are worth the trade-off. But in the quest for maximum physical fitness, you shouldn't have to sacrifice any one aspect of physical health, not even one strand of hair.

When you're offered a supplement or steroids or the latest fad workout, question it. Always research something before you "just do it." "Everybody else is doing it" is not a valid reason. You're body is unique and most of the joy of exercise is in finding your own path to fitness. In the following chapters, we're going to talk about the basic facts of exercise—about how muscles function and interrelate—so that if a workout or a supplement promises that X is going to happen, you'll be able to know otherwise. Stopping and asking, "What exactly is this going to do for me," and taking the time and energy to find out for yourself slows down the process. And that's OK—fitness is a lifelong process, not something that's subject to quick fixes.

Maximizing your fitness is something that you should do as part of your everyday lifestyle. You can push yourself to a momentary extreme, push yourself to new levels of achievement—but the way in which you go about it needs to be a concerted, fact-based process. If somebody comes along promising you all these great things in 30 days or less, then you know — as anyone should— that you're being sold something akin to a very large bridge.

Do your own homework. Spend the time and effort. Logic dictates that if you can get it today, then it probably could be gone tomorrow. But if you do it right, it'll be here for a lifetime. And that's what extreme fitness is all about. Life is, after all, the ultimate extreme sport.

VARY YOUR ROUTINE

My first understanding of body alignment, balance, and biomechanics came when I studied dance over the summers during college. I studied modern dance, ballet, tap, and jazz dancing. My desire to create the kind of body that I always wanted led me to pursue training that seems light years away from my football player-weight lifter-bodybuilder background. Talk about blazing your own path!

People ask me, "Is the answer to perfect fitness spinning? Is it in-line skating? Is the answer in step aerobics?" This is the wrong attitude. Maintaining lifelong fitness and reaching your physical potential involve keeping your body and mind challenged. It means doing, first, what you enjoy doing, and then adding new things— creating your own path to personal fitness.

So how did I end up dancing? When I was a freshman in college, I took a speech class with a professor who was also the theatre director. He thought I had some performing potential, but he knew that I was playing football at the time. (This was in a time when jocks were jocks and everybody else was everybody else.) My professor was very persistent about combining my physicality and verbal skills, so he got me to audition for a physically demanding role in a play. During the play, I met an actress who ran a dance studio. She convinced me to take some classes and helped me appreciate the athleticism in dance, especially among dancers like Gene Kelly (who was quite an athlete).

Naturally, I got a lot of flak from my football buddies for taking dance— until an athletic consultant suggested the entire team take modern dance. The application, though, was totally different. The dance was presented as a kind of workout; the players were taught only what they could apply to their sport. Meanwhile, I studied dance for the sake of learning dance—I wanted to get all I could out of it. I find that there are innumerable benefits from learning a discipline entirely and not just piecemeal.

For instance, a lot of gyms offer "power yoga." It's all about the workout; the instructor doesn't talk about the whole philosophy of yoga. I say, if you're going to do yoga, do it right—go to a yoga center. That way you'll get all the benefits out of it. So often people say, "Well, if I'm just looking for the physical benefits, why do I need to learn the mental skills and the meditation?" I'll tell you something that we'll discuss more later: the mind controls the muscles. The best athletes use their brains as much as their brawn to succeed. Don't ignore the mental aspect of a physical discipline!

Martial arts is a discipline, yoga is a discipline, ballet is a discipline. To really get something useful from each of these, you need to dedicate yourself to that art form or physical technique. If you simply throw a yoga "workout" or a ballet "workout" into an aerobics class setting, you're going to get a watered-down version of the real discipline.

When I threw myself into each discipline, I completely dedicated myself to it. To others, it may have seemed that playing football and studying ballet was going from one extreme to the other. But I was exploring my physicality, challenging my body, and always learning.

Eventually I got to the point where I got more out of the training than I did out of the sport that I was training for. I was so rewarded by the ability to change my body and make it respond, that I determined that ultimately, this—working out—was my sport. In a sense, I was my own sport. If I wanted to play football or dance or play golf (my current passion), I *became* my own sport. I could train my body so that it could adapt to any discipline.

There's a reward in discovering the joy of exercise and the joy of your own physicality through many different sports and disciplines. You should take your own path and not blindly follow some universal exercise regime. But to keep yourself fit enough to excel at your favorite physical pastime, as well as pursue some new sports that intrigue you, and even move onto more extreme levels of exercise, you need to maintain a base level of fitness that your current workout may not be providing you with. Exactly how you maintain your base level is totally up to you, but you can't do it without understanding exactly what muscles to train, why, and how. This book will explain those things and offer exercise options so that you can create your own workout and mix it up when you need a new challenge.

There's no one best way to physical fitness—create your own path and master your own extremes.

EXERCISE 101:
A REFRESHER COURSE
FOR THE
FIT-BUT-FRUSTRATED

AT THE GYM WHERE I WORK, I often see people spending up to an hour and a half on the treadmill. Like a policeman confronting a jumper on a roof, I have to carefully coax these people off the equipment. I tell them, "More is just more; more isn't necessarily better."

Failure to grasp this concept has stalled more athletes at the intermediate level than you can imagine. I'll say it again: *More is just more; more isn't necessarily better!*

Your body's job is to adapt to stress. It will adapt to become as efficient at a certain movement as possible. Once it does that, it stops adapting. It stops changing. It has figured out how to perform the exercise using the least amount of energy (which may be frustrating if you're trying to get it to shed that last 10 pounds of fat). Regardless of whether or not you keep going another five or 10 or 30 minutes on the treadmill, your body has already maximized its efficiency. More of the same exercise isn't challenging it. Once it adapts totally to the specific exercise, the effectiveness of that exercise lessens— even as you're spending more and more time doing it.

Less really *is* more, because once your body has maximized its efficiency in performing a certain exercise, it provides more strength or speed or distance with less overall effort. That's how the body *wants* to work. But too often we try to force our own individual will: "I've got to stay on this treadmill for an hour to make my body do what I want it to do!" What we don't realize is that we're just wasting our time.

So if you're one of those folks whose whole workout involves spending an hour on the treadmill or the StairMaster, I suggest you slow down and stop. Maybe when you started out you couldn't even do 15 minutes. And then you could do 30 and then 45. And if 45 is good, you reasoned, then an hour must be even better. But after you reached that hour— and were doing it five or six days a week for weeks at a time—your body stopped responding. Still, you keep doing the same thing but expecting change (which, by the way, is the definition of insanity).

The first rule of training, therefore, is to vary your routine when your body stops responding, i.e., adapting. Keep giving it new challenges. Sometimes that can be as simple as changing the order of the exercises you do; sometimes it may require changing the exercises themselves. Just remember, at a certain point (which we'll discuss later) merely doing more push-ups or dumbbell presses or minutes on the treadmill isn't going to improve your fitness level.

THE MEASURE OF FITNESS

Hanging onto "beginner-level" concepts also holds intermediate-level athletes back from progressing to the next level. For example, most beginners judge their fitness level by the bathroom scale. But that tells a person only his or her total amount of weight. It doesn't indicate how much of that weight is fat, how much is muscle, and how much is bone. The scale, therefore, can give beginners a gross misconception about how fit they are. Especially as beginners start exercising, they begin to metabolize more lean muscle tissue, which is more dense than fat and carries more weight per pound.

When I train "scale-conscious" beginners, they often freak out after a week or two and say, "I came here to lose weight, and I've *gained* weight! You don't know what you're doing. I'm going back to my treadmill!" I have to explain that initially, weight gain occurs because muscles are developing faster than fat is burning off—but that doesn't mean that fat isn't burning off at all. It just takes a little more time.

So when a beginner sees that scale go up even though she's working out, she shouldn't get upset. She, like every other serious exerciser, has to find other ways to monitor her progress.

First—and this may not be the quantitative measurement most people are looking for—the person working out consistently is going to *feel better*. He's going to experience a sense of euphoria, confidence, or greater strength and power. He'll feel much more energetic.

The second qualitative, as opposed to quantitative, measure of fitness is hearing people say things like, "Did you lose weight?" In fact, the person may know he's gained weight—in terms of muscle density—but people will notice his weight is distributed differently. Muscle has a shape, a definition, which takes up less space than flab.

The next measure is how the person's clothes fit. A woman's dress size may be the same, but the garment will "hang" differently on her. A man may have dropped a waist size; his pants may feel too loose.

The final qualitative measure will be when the person can stand naked in front of a mirror and actually see noticeable changes. He may say, "Wow, my waist is smaller! Look at my chest, look at my legs, look at my butt — it's lifted back up again! Is that possible?" Yes, it is.

That point may come in eight weeks, eight months, or two years. Everybody's different. But in my experience, when my clients reach that stage, they say, "I threw my scale away — what do I care how much I weigh? It's how I look and feel—that's how I judge my fitness."

So if you've been exercising regularly for several years, and you're still judging your fitness by the bathroom scale, give it up! It's time to move beyond weight goals and toward total health goals.

For a more quantitative measure of fitness, you can spend a lot of money at health centers having your BMI—Body Mass Index—precisely calculated. But you don't need to do that. Focus on how you feel and how you look—that's the best measure of fitness.

No matter what your sport or favorite physical activity, reaching your peak physical performance for it means training on three fronts: flexibility, cardio-vascular capacity, and strength. Let's take an in-depth look at each of these areas.

STRETCH YOURSELF

There's a resurgent interest in stretching these days. The good news is that stretching prevents injuries and promotes flexibility. The bad news is that most people are doing the old, traditional stretches like bending over and touching the toes. A stretch like that puts more pressure on the lower back and, over time, can cause damage. I'm not bad-mouthing stretching in general, but if you end up doing more harm than good, what's the sense of doing it? While stretching, you should know *why* you're stretching—what the purpose of stretching is—and how to do it to achieve that purpose.

The first thing to realize is that *stretching does not constitute a warm-up*, as so many even long-time exercisers believe. You need to warm up your muscles *even before you stretch*. I said that to a client the other day and she looked at me like I had three heads. I made an analogy for her: Think of the muscles you're stretching as a rubber band. First, you know you can stretch that rubber band only so far. Now put the rubber band in the freezer. It's going to snap much sooner than if you had put it in warm water. The warmer the rubber, the more elastic it is. Your muscles are similar to that rubber band—you need to warm them up before you stretch them out. Warmth is a function of blood flow. Increase the blood flow to your muscles, and the "warmer"

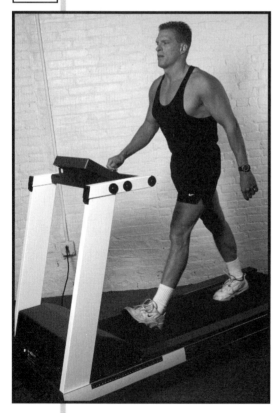
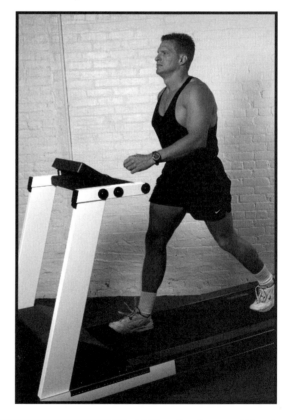

they become. When you begin to stretch, your muscle fibers are given a signal to separate, to move in opposite directions. But if they're not warmed up, they will actually do just the opposite as a protective measure. They'll actually tighten up and work against you.

You may try to go in one direction and your body may respond by trying to go the other direction. The muscle contraction is a survival mechanism — the muscle doesn't know you *intend* to do the stretch; it is afraid that its connective fibers are going to be completely separated.

If you continue to force the stretch, the muscle fibers will eventually separate. But, by this point you have already caused an injury inside the muscle fibers even before you started your first exercise. That may be why you are sore later—even though you don't feel sore at the time.

However, if you warm up your muscles with a little walking or light biking—something that's not likely to traumatize muscles but will let them know, hey, we're going to do some work now—your muscles will be more relaxed and willing to stretch. Warming up first also increases blood flow to the muscles and releases synovial fluid, which is like a lubricant for the joints.

When you're ready to stretch, remember our primary concept: A little is a lot. Stretch to the point where you feel slight tension. Hold it there for 10 to 15 seconds; don't push it. Then repeat the stretch.

WHEN TO STRETCH. When I work out, I don't do all my stretches at once. There's nothing wrong with doing them that way; I just prefer to incorporate stretching in between sets of my strength training exercises. I feel it helps to increase the blood flow in between sets of each exercise I'm doing. Increasing blood flow allows for oxygenated blood to be carried into that muscle, and toxins to be carried out, so that the muscle's ready to go onto the next set. Some people, however, prefer to stretch after they work out, to help cool down their muscles and ensure that they don't tighten up right after exercising. The only rule concerning when to stretch is this: *stretch after you've warmed up.* Stretching does *not* constitute a warm-up.

Most people think that big muscles are tight, tense muscles, when in fact the opposite is true. Weak muscles are tight muscles. An inflexible muscle, or tight muscle, is actually an underdeveloped muscle. Strength training alone can increase that muscle's flexibility. What's more, stretching can actually make tight, weak muscles stronger. Part of the reason for that has to do with the nerves inside the muscle sending certain signals, and part has to do with

19

the fact that just by stretching, you're using muscles that may not otherwise get much use. A strong muscle is a supple muscle. It's a self-supporting superstructure.

TYPES OF STRETCHES. Now you know why to stretch and when to stretch. What about how to stretch? I'll describe basic stretches for each of the major muscle groups in Chapter 4. But you might want to know that there are different styles of stretching—assisted stretching, ballistic stretching, and static stretching.

Most people do "static" stretches. You assume one position, move into a stretch position, hold the stretch, then release. Unaware of how to position their bodies correctly before and during the stretch, though, most people will hold a stretch too long in a biomechanically incorrect position. They end up not stretching the intended muscle at all. They believe they need to really "feel" the stretch, which usually means that they're stretching into the ligaments and tendons of the joints. Unlike muscles, however, ligaments and tendons stay stretched—they do not regain their rigidity. They're like the elastic waistband on your favorite pair of sweatpants—once that band has been stretched too far, it doesn't snap back. *You do not want to stretch ligaments and tendons*—they do not repair. Positioning your body correctly and maintaining proper form during the stretch are essential to improving flexibility. (Chapter 4 will describe stretches in detail.)

Ballistic stretching is also called dynamic stretching. The body stays in motion, moving from one stretch into the next, then repeating. People doing this kind of stretching must be careful not to "bounce" into their stretches, but maintain smooth, fluid movements. Ballistic stretching routines are usually designed to mirror the kinds of movements the person is likely to do during a particular sport.

HOLD IT. The muscle's ability to hold the tension of a stretch dissipates after about 10 to 15 seconds. If you keep trying to force it, that tension will move into the joint — and you run the risk of injury. You may not feel the injury while you're stretching, but just get out onto the soccer field or tennis court and you will.

BREATHE! One thing most people take for granted is knowing how to breathe, but you'd be surprised how many people I've met in the gym who seem to forget when they start to exercise. The mantra for stretching—and for any kind of physical exertion—is "exhale on execution; inhale on preparation." In other words, as you execute the movement, exhale, and as you prepare to return and start the next movement, inhale.

That rule can be a little cumbersome for some people to remember, so I tell my clients, "Just breathe." Half my clients will be huffing and puffing, exaggerating their breathing because they're so focused on it. And the others are completely silent. I tell them, "You're not breathing." When you're just starting to exercise, there are so many things to keep in mind to make sure you're stretching technically correctly, probably the last thing you're going to be thinking about is your breathing. Having a trainer or even a friend there to monitor your breathing for a workout or two can be very helpful.

The famous "grunters" in professional tennis, like Monica Seles and the Williams sisters, are examples of good breathers. Tennis coaches tell their young students to exhale when they hit the ball, i.e., at execution, and to make sure the students are doing it, they tell them to make a sound. Over time, making this sound becomes a habit.

I had one client who was getting nauseous whenever he worked out. Even though he was getting into shape, physically improving, he always seemed to hyperventilate. I realized he was breathing in and out of his mouth as opposed to in through his nose and out through his mouth. Your body works very efficiently that way — inhalation through the nostrils and exhalation through the mouth. If you breathe both in through and out of your mouth, you're likely to get dry mouth and suffer an imbalance in how much air you're taking in and how much you're letting out. My client was getting nauseous because the nitrogen levels in his blood were building up. He got better immediately once he started breathing correctly.

Stretching and breathing correctly, which may seem simple enough, are serious business. They can affect your energy level, your susceptibility to injury, and hence your ability to then continue exercising.

PUT YOUR HEART INTO IT

We need to define some terms. People tend to use "cardio training" and "aerobic training" interchangeably. Technically, they're not the same.

Cardiovascular training refers to training the most important muscle in

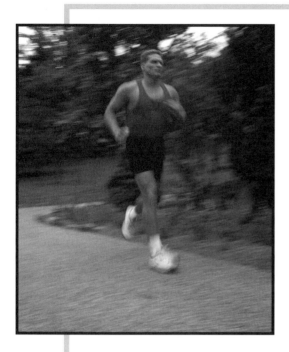
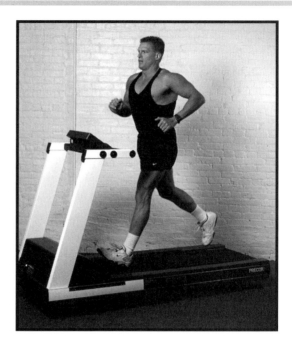

your body—your heart. "Cardio" actually means "heart." So "cardio training" is heart training in which you try to get your heart to pump blood more efficiently. Instead of beating at, say, 110 beats per minute (bpm) to accomplish a certain exercise, cardio training eventually brings your heart rate down to 70 bpm while performing the same task. You're doing the same exercise, but your heart is working more efficiently, beating fewer times to accomplish the same task.

"Aerobic" refers to oxygen. When you're doing "aerobic" activity, your body is primarily using oxygen as an energy source. When you're doing "anaerobic" exercise, like weight training, you're using the glycogen stored in the muscle cells instead of oxygen. You can, however, get a cardiovascular benefit from anaerobic training like lifting weights. For example, you can do a free-standing squat, which trains your gluteal (butt) and leg muscles by using your own body weight as resistance. That's an anaerobic activity because your muscles are tapping their glycogen stores for energy. Do one squat and you may feel it in your muscles, but you're not exactly huffing and puffing. Now do 15 reps. Now do two sets of 15 reps. Your heart is definitely thumping now!

It's the combination of anaerobic and aerobic activity that provides the best cardio training.

SUDDEN IMPACT. People think the term "high-impact aerobics" connotes "high-level benefits," as opposed to "low-impact" exercise. "High-impact" anything doesn't necessarily mean better—in fact, it can mean worse. "Impact" refers to the amount of pressure your subjecting your joints to. All that jumping up and down in aerobics class gets your heart going, but it can also do a number on your knees. Low-impact resistance training, done correctly of course, doesn't put as much strain on your joints. That's not to say that one type of exercise is better than the other—in fact, the ideal is the combination of the two.

MONITOR YOUR CARDIO CAPACITY. There have been some very good technological advances in the heart rate monitors that you can buy in stores now, like the Polar brand. Certain gym machines, like Life Fitness Equipment, have built-in monitors so you can watch your heart rate as you jog on the treadmill. People who prefer running or biking outdoors can simply take their pulse, either at the wrist or the carotid (neck) artery for 10 seconds, and multiply the pulse count by six to get their beats per minute.

You should try to train at your target heart rate, which is 70 to 80 percent of your maximum heart rate. To determine your maximum heart rate (MHR), subtract your age from 220. To determine your target heart rate (THR), multiply your MHR by .70 (for 70 percent intensity) and .80 (for 80 percent intensity). Here is an example for a 35 year old:

MHR = 220 − 35 = 185 beats per minute
THR (70% intensity) = 185 × .70 = 130 beats per minute
THR (80% intensity) = 185 × .80 = 148 beats per minute

HOW MUCH CARDIO DO YOU NEED? A well-balanced fitness program, according to the American College of Sports Medicine, includes 30 minutes of cardiovascular exercise three times a week. Naturally, if you're training for a marathon, your goals are going to be a little different. But if you're working out in order to achieve overall peak fitness or maximum performance for a particular sport, make sure you have 30 minutes of cardio activity three times a week. More than that is probably a waste of time.

Another important thing to remember is that cardio training doesn't just mean running. There's biking, jumping rope, aerobics class, dance class—don't let yourself get bored.

INTENSIFY. One way to make a 30-minute cardio workout more intense is to try "interval training." Interval training is simply doing a variety of different modes of cardiovascular aerobic activity at different intensities for different durations. For example, say you pick a treadmill, a stationary bike, a StairMaster, and then a rowing machine. You'd spend approximately seven minutes on each piece of equipment and vary the intensity—e.g., jog for two minutes, run hard for two minutes, jog for three minutes, etc. You would, in fact, burn more calories because your body would have to shift slightly to accommodate each intensity and each exercise while maintaining its energy supply.

You don't even have to switch equipment—just intensities. In fact, you don't have to use equipment at all—just go outside. Run up a hill instead of along a flat path. Create your own program.

A lot of treadmills offer different program settings—the heart rate program, the fat-burner program, etc. "How about doing 'The Sally Jo Program?'" I said to a client. "That's not on here, " she said. "Sure it is. You've got a button called 'manual.'"

Put the machine on a manual setting. Now you have the freedom to control the intensity of that activity — increase the speed or the incline.

People get bored out of their minds in the gym because they're spending hours on the treadmill. That's why equipment manufacturers install TVs, videos, and even Internet access on their machines. But you don't need to spend an hour doing the same old thing. All you need is 30 minutes—and an imagination to mix it up.

STRONG MEDICINE

There was a time when most people thought of strength training as body-building. But today even golfers and marathon runners include strength workouts in their training programs.

The truth is, no matter what your sport or physical fitness goals, strength training plays an integral part. Your body develops its agility and coordination through its musculature. That doesn't mean your muscles have to be enormous to achieve your particular goals; in fact, basic strength training exercises won't make them enormous. But basic weight (or "resistance") training will develop your muscles so they can adapt to the different physical stresses you place on your body. Your ability to have a sudden burst of energy without injuring yourself, your ability to pick up a sport you may not have played for 20 years and perform at your peak, your ability to maintain bone density as you age . . . strength training makes these possible.

SPOT TRAINING. Some people think they've got to train in a specific way for their sport — for instance, training just their legs if they're skiers or training just their upper bodies for football. Sport-specific training became very popular a few years ago, and it's true that for the elite world-class athlete, targeted training may work well. But unless you're a professional athlete and can afford to sacrifice well-balanced fitness on the days you're *not* competing, I say stick with a holistic, total body workout.

Ask yourself what your body is doing the majority of the time. How do you make your living? Do you want to train specifically for an activity you do only a small percentage of the time, or do you want to train for maximum fitness for the rest of your life?

Train for what you do the majority of time. You will then have more energy and strength not only for everyday activities, but for the athletic activities you enjoy as well.

One day I was walking the gym floor and saw a woman in her middle to late 50s, who seemed in fairly good shape. She was sitting at the end of a bench with no more than a five pound dumbbell in her hand, rotating and twisting her wrist while resting her forearm on her knee. It looked as though she was trying to strengthen her wrist and forearm.

I observed her for a couple of minutes and noticed that in between each set she would stop and knead the area in and around her elbow. She had done this to such an extent that here forearm was red from the friction where she'd been rubbing it, which told me that she was in pain — whether self-imposed or otherwise.

I walked over and introduced myself. She proceeded to tell me that she thought she had tendonitis. I said, "How are you trying to train your muscle — what are you trying to train it for?"

"I incurred this injury last year playing golf," she said. "My golf pro said I had trouble with my grip strength, that I needed to grip the club harder."

(As a golfer myself, I knew you're not supposed to grip the club harder; you're supposed to hold it loosely but firmly.)

She said, "I figured that if I did this spot workout to this one area, then I'd be able to develop the muscles there and then do what the pro told me I was supposed to do."

Her intentions were honorable, but she had too much zeal. She thought that kneading the body part would help, when in fact it was causing the inflammation and redness. What's more, she was neglecting to work out her supporting muscles—her biceps, triceps, and shoulder muscles, all of which are integral in executing a good golf swing. She was a prime candidate to develop muscle imbalances that could lead to serious injuries either on or off the golf course.

The funny part of this story is, whom do you think she was playing against, whom do you think she was trying to keep up with? You might think maybe one of her children. But she was trying to keep up with her mom and dad, who were in their 80s and playing golf four times a week. She'd worn out her arm trying to keep up with her parents!

The problem with sports-specific training is that often people try to concentrate on one area and fail to train the surrounding — and supporting— muscles. This is as common a problem with intermediate-level athletes as

Remember the Basics

- Always warm up with five to ten minutes of light cardio activity before stretching or strength training.
- Hold stretches no more or less than 10 to 15 seconds.
- Exhale on execution; inhale on preparation.
- Breathe in through the nose and out through the mouth.
- Work out *all* your major muscles; avoid "spot" training.
- Own it before you load it.
- Never strength train the same muscle groups two days in a row; strength train no more than three days a week.
- Vary your routine when your body stops adapting.
- Recognize when more is just more, when more is not necessarily better.

with beginners. When one muscle becomes overdeveloped and its opposite and supporting muscle becomes underdeveloped, you have a prime situation for injury. This often happens when people want to train, say, their forearms, but they totally ignore the larger muscles of the body—their legs and back muscles, for example. These muscles help your smaller muscles do their jobs, so they need to be trained in conjunction with the smaller ones.

Furthermore, while a sport may demand strength from a particular muscle group, like the arms, most sports require your body to engage many different muscle groups at one time. In other words, you need to be able to twist and turn your body in order to hit shots or maintain balance. This motion is tough on your spine, unless you have strong and stable muscles surrounding it. And you can't have strong, injury-resistant back muscles unless you have strong abdominal muscles. Training your abs and back muscles is known as "core training," and it is essential to any kind of workout program.

To reiterate, the biggest risk with spot training is muscle imbalance: over-training some muscles and undertraining others. This can lead to serious injury, even though you may feel like you're in good shape. The exercises presented in the next chapter are designed to provide you with a well-balanced, thorough workout.

HOW DO MUSCLES ACTUALLY GROW? Hormones account for a lot, which is why men have greater potential for larger muscles than women. Many women, in fact, shy away from strength training because they worry that their muscles will become "big" in a physically unattractive, unfeminine way. True, their muscles will become conditioned (a.k.a. toned), but unless they start taking hormones or are genetically predisposed, women will not get huge muscles from basic strength training.

In addition to responding to hormonal influences, muscles grow when their cells divide and multiply in response to an injury. A major injury, of course, would defeat the purpose of training. But when you're training safely, you're still creating little "microtraumas" to the muscle. When you rest, the body repairs those microtraumas and the area becomes stronger as a result. This strengthening process depends on two things: giving yourself enough time to rest and repair (which means never training the same muscles two days in a row) and not allowing microtraumas to become macrotraumas by overtraining in other ways, such as using too heavy a weight.

So keep to a schedule. Never strength train any muscle group two consecutive days, even if you don't feel sore or fatigued. You can't feel the microtraumas that are healing on a microscopic level.

Sure, in the past, East German and Soviet Olympic coaches trained their athletes every day, but they also drugged their athletes, gave them sports massages every few hours, and took biopsies of their muscle tissues. We're talking about a government-instituted experiment in which athletes had their own scientists following them around. Trust me, if you start training like that, you'll need paramedics following you around.

Ask yourself what your strength goals are. Do you want large muscles to achieve a particular physique or to perform a certain strength-intensive activity? Or do you want to remain relatively lean, yet strong?

If your goal is to build as much muscle as possible, you may ask, what does it take for the body to metabolize one pound of muscle? It takes 3,500 calories a week; when divided over seven days, that means taking in an extra 500 calories a day, preferably in the form of protein. In other words, at *best* you could expect to metabolize one pound of muscle a week. Believing ads that promise more than that is unrealistic, and you can do more harm than good trying to develop more.

THE MAJOR MUSCLE GROUPS. There are three major areas of the body that you need to be concerned with when you strength train: lower body, upper body, and core muscles. Always start with the largest muscles first because they're the primary "movers." We're bipeds, so our largest muscles, the ones that move us through life, are our leg muscles. The first group of muscles to train, therefore, are the quadriceps, which are on the fronts of the thighs. Adjoining their movement are the hip flexor muscles.

The second group of muscles to train are the supporting leg muscles, the hamstrings, which are on the backs of the thighs. Their adjoining muscles are the gluteal, or butt, muscles.

The smaller, though still important, lower body muscles are the inner thigh muscles known as the adductors and abductors, as well as the calves (gastrocnemius) and shin (tibialis anterior) muscles.

Often times at the gym, I'll ask my clients whether they've worked out their leg muscles. They'll say, "I did my legs when I warmed up on the treadmill, so I don't need to train them anymore."

Training all those large leg muscles simultaneously has the single greatest physiological effect on your entire cardiovascular system, which is why so much cardio exercise involves using your legs—running, biking, etc. But when you use the muscles one at a time, it challenges you body in ways it's not used to. Your leg muscles *are used* to working together in the most efficient manner to propel you down the sidewalk. How can you challenge them to do something they're *not* used to doing? Train them individually.

In Chapter 4, I'm going to show you how to perform a freestanding squat with no additional resistance. Your own body weight and gravity will work against you. If all you've been doing to train your legs is running, you'll be surprised how much you "feel" a couple sets of squats! You may think you've never used your legs before.

The second largest group of muscles to train are in your torso. Your abs are responsible for spinal flexion and your lower back muscles are responsible for spinal extension. These are your "core" muscles. Weakness here accounts for more backaches and injuries than accidents do.

When I was a bodybuilder, how strong my abs actually were had nothing to do with my success in the sport. I was judged on how well these muscles looked. I got them to show by getting my body fat and my fluid levels as low as humanly possible. It didn't matter what I could *do* with my abs; it mattered that you could *see* them.

What obscures muscles is body fat. (By the way, fat doesn't become muscle and muscle doesn't become fat.) Fat is the obscuring layer on top of our existing muscle structure. And people can have a lot of obstruction and still have very conditioned muscles. There are some elite athletes at the top of their games, primarily baseball players and golfers, to whom you might be tempted to say, "Well, you don't *look* like much of an athlete!" They don't necessarily have to have "lean" muscular structures, but they certainly have some pretty strong muscles maintaining the integrity of their spines.

So figure out what your goal is in terms of training your core muscles. Do you care whether your abs show? Or is functionality your only concern?

The third largest muscle group to train is the upper body muscles: the pectoral (chest) muscles of the front and the deltoids, latissimus dorsi, and trapezius (upper back and shoulder muscles) of the back. These muscles support and adjoin the smaller arm muscles—the biceps (front) and triceps (back).

When training these muscles, I usually employ the push-pull method, alternating exercises for the extension muscles (extensors) with those for flexion muscles (flexors). This gives us the following order: First you train your

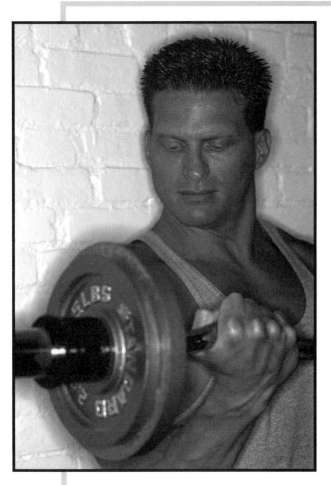

pecs, then your lats, then your delts and traps, and finally your biceps and triceps. Working from largest to smallest and front to back helps prevent injury.

Most people tend to train what they like and what responds, which depends on individual genetics. Some people, therefore, might just train their arms and their legs because that's what looks good to them. Ironically, people tend to work on their strengths, not necessarily on their weaknesses. But ignoring your weaknesses can set you up for trouble.

Men, for instance, tend to work the "show" muscles, which are the upper body muscles— chest, biceps—and neglect their legs. Women are just the opposite. They're much more lower-body conscious and neglect the upper body. Pretty much everyone across the board — old, young, man, woman — is very conscious of the abs.

One of my new clients is a young guy who had been training before he came to me. I questioned him about his exercise history, and he told me that he'd been working out for a while. I could tell he was no beginner, but he was no athlete either. The first workout I put him through was a total body workout — lower body, core, and upper body. I didn't concentrate on any one area; I just made sure he got a thorough workout. Afterwards, he seemed to be excited and scheduled another appointment right away.

But he didn't show up for it. He cancelled and made excuses the next time, too. He finally confessed to me that he was afraid to come back to the gym. As most of the people in the gym were not in as good shape as he was, I was baffled. Then he complained of extreme soreness after our first workout. I asked him for details. It really didn't make sense to me. Then it dawned on me. Everything that was sore was literally behind him. His sore muscles were his back, his butt, his hamstrings, and his calves. Everything on the back half of his body hurt, but nothing on the front of his body hurt. He had never thought to train his back muscles. "Brad," he said, "if I couldn't see it, I didn't train it."

"Front" and "back" muscles are also called "extensors" and "flexors" or "agonist" and "antagonist" muscles. While one muscle is flexing, the other is extending; while one is contracting, the other is stretching. Properly training both prevents dangerous imbalances.

For instance, a heavy-set woman walked up to me at the gym the other day. She said, "I think I'm getting shin splints when I walk on the treadmill," and she pointed to her shins. "What should I do?"

My jaw dropped when I looked at her legs. I said, "Do you know that you have world-class bodybuilder calves?" She had the biggest, hardest, most muscular calves I'd ever seen on a woman. Yet overall, she was 50 to 60 pounds overweight.

She said, "Yeah, I know—I've never done calf exercises a day in my life. I got them from my dad."

I said, "Yeah, I can see that. I mean no offense, but there's no way you could have trained to get those."

Because her calves were so overdeveloped, her tibialis anterior, which is the muscle down the front of the shin, was underdeveloped and tight —that's why it was causing her pain. I showed her how to do toe raises to build strength in the muscles of the front of her leg—and she was off and running again.

CHOOSING A WEIGHT. Before you pick up the heaviest weight around, remember this rule: You need to "own it before you load it." In other words, you must be able to do the exercise correctly, using the most efficient form, before you even think about adding weight.

Once you add resistance to a movement, everything changes. You are prone to perform the exercise incorrectly and that can lead to injury. For example, stand straight with good posture and your arms at your sides, then lift your hands up to your shoulders. Now perform the same motion, only holding ten pound dumbbells in each hand. You will be prone to arch your back, allowing it to "help" your arm lift the weight. This movement misses the point of the exercise—you're no longer training your arms, and you could be hurting your back!

Your body, by its very nature, wants to take the path of least resistance. The goal of resistance training, therefore, is to make the path of least resistance primarily muscular—not skeletal or joint-related. Over the long run, bones and joints wear out, and they do not repair themselves the way muscles do.

When I walk around a gym, I'm horrified to see how some people's form is actually doing them more harm than good. They are developing poor posture that might someday cripple them.

For example, many people think a squat involves bending from the knees, but that's a deep knee-bend. And deep knee-bends wear out your knees.

I was recently training a woman on the proper squat movement, which involves more of your hips than your knees. She finally got the form right and could do a couple sets. So then I asked her to do a proper squat holding a ten-pound dumbbell between her legs— just to hold onto a dumbbell in her hands and continue to do what she'd done for several weeks. She couldn't do it.

In the next chapter, I'll discuss when to add repetitions to an exercise, when to add weight, and how much weight to add as you progress. I'll also talk about varying your exercises to create a workout program that will keep you challenged.

The fact is, physical changes that happen as a result of exercise—fat loss revealing muscle shape—occur most dramatically when someone who hasn't exercised in a while—"Joe Deconditioned"—first starts out on an exercise program. The problem is, Joe expects that initial rate of improvement to continue. He gets frustrated when he doesn't see progress even though he thinks he's working out harder and longer. His body seems to come to a complete halt—proving the old adage that the last five pounds are the hardest to lose.

If that's happened to you, now's the time to question the way you're exercising. The same exercises done in the same way will stop producing changes. Your body adapts. Just adding more—more reps, more time on the treadmill—will do no good. You need to mix up your routine and keep your body adapting.

THE ART OF CREATING A WORKOUT TAILORED FOR YOUR BODY

IN A COUPLE OF PAGES you're going to see a table that includes each of the muscle groups and the corresponding stretches and exercises you can do to target each muscle group. In addition, two levels of intensity—in terms of sets and reps—for each exercise are given. The strength training exercises are varied so that you can use your own body weight as resistance, use free weights, or use standard gym equipment, depending on how you prefer to train—and for variations on the central themes of extreme training.

Before you start to train, create a workout schedule. Perhaps you want to strength train on Mondays, Wednesdays, and Fridays, and do 30 minutes of cardio activity Tuesdays, Thursdays, and Saturdays. Maybe you want to combine your cardio training and strength training workouts on the same days. However you carve up your training schedule, always remember to warm up with five to ten minutes of light cardio activity first, and stretch at some point thereafter.

Chapter 4 will illustrate and describe how to perform each exercise properly and safely. I'll even show you typical "bad form" for each of the exercises so you'll know what *not* to do. Breaking bad habits is especially difficult for intermediate-level athletes, but doing so is crucial if you want to move on to the next level.

The Extreme Training Workout assumes you have achieved a certain base fitness level and can do the following with little trouble:

MEN	WOMEN
Bench press at least 185 lbs., 8 to 10 reps.	Bench press at least 50 lbs.
Do 100 crunches.	Do 100 crunches.
Jog 3.5 miles in 30 minutes.	Jog 3 miles in 30 minutes.

(If you have trouble doing the above, you can still do the Extreme Workout, but do only those exercises that use your own body weight as resistance before you start adding free weights, and begin with two sets of 12 reps for each exercise. Slowly build up to Level II.)

Start out at Level II (intermediate) on the table. Once you can complete three or four sets with a moderate weight, you can increase the weight—and lower the reps. *Increase your sets from three to four before you increase the weight.* In other words, if doing three sets of dumbbell presses with a ten-pound weight is no longer challenging, add a fourth set before you add another five pounds to the weight. Add repetitions to increase the intensity first, and once you can handle that weight so that the maximum number of sets and reps is no longer taxing you, only then move up in weight (adding no more than five pounds at a time). When you decide to move on to Level III, you may want to decrease the amount of weight you're using at first.

Ultimately you want to develop a repertoire of exercises. So mix up your workout—don't always do squats, for instance, when working out your legs—try the leg presses and the deadlifts. That way, you will be creating your own workout based on what is most challenging to you.

You may find that you already do many of the exercises listed here. But you probably don't do them the same way I describe—in fact, you may be doing them wrong (i.e., inefficiently and injuriously). It may be hard to break bad habits at your stage, but it's very important to learn to do the exercises correctly. You may even find your body is responding to the correct form like a beginner's body would. Don't lose your motivation—stick with it and work through the exercises correctly!

It takes a consistency of effort over a period of time, doing these exercises precisely, to train your body so that it is almost incapable of doing them incorrectly. If an exercise is safe, it's effective; and if it's effective, it's always safe.

SAFETY + EFFECTIVENESS = MAXIMUM INTENSITY = RESULTS

MUSCLE GROUPS	STRETCHES	EXERCISES	LEVEL II (Intermediate)	LEVEL III (Advanced)
LEGS/BUTT:			3–4 sets x 12–15 reps	4 sets x 15–20 reps
Quadriceps	Quad stretch	Athletic squats		
Glutes	Glute stretches (2)	Or: One-legged squats		
Abductors/Adductors	Inner thigh stretch	Ballet squats		
Hamstrings	Hamstring stretch	Flexed deadlifts		
Calves	Calf stretch	One-leg leg presses		
		Calf raises		
ABS AND LOWER BACK:			2–3 supersets* x 20–30 reps	3–4 supersets x 30–50 reps
Abdominals	Knee hug	Basic crunches		
Rectus Abdominus	Back extensions (3)	Advanced crunches		
Obliques	Cat stretch	Reverse crunches		
Erector Spinae				
CHEST:			3–4 sets x 10–12 reps	4 sets x 8–10 reps
Pectoralis Major	Standing pec stretch	Push-ups		
		Or: Incline bench presses		
		Dumbbell presses		
		Bench push-ups		
		Standing cable flyes		
UPPER BACK:			3–4 sets x 12–15 reps	4 sets x 8–10 reps
Latissimus Dorsi	Lat stretch	Pull-ups		
		Single-arm dumbbell rows		
		Or: Reverse-grip pull-downs		
		Straight-arm lat pull-downs		
SHOULDERS AND UPPER BACK:			3 sets x 12–15 reps	4 sets x 10–12 reps
Deltoids	Shoulder stretch	Barbell clean-presses		
Trapezius	Neck stretch	Or: Seated dumbbell presses		
		Dumbbell lateral raises		
		Or: Bent-over rear delt raises		
ARMS (FRONT):			3 sets x 12–15 reps	3–4 sets x 10–12 reps
Biceps	Bicep stretch	Standing barbell curls		
		Alternating dumbbell curls		
		Or: Hammer curls		
		Cable bicep curls		
ARMS (BACK):			3 sets x 12–15 reps	3–4 sets x 10–12 reps
Triceps	Tricep stretch	Bench dips		
		Overhead dumbbell extensions		
		Or: Dumbbell kickbacks		
		Cable tricep extensions		
Forearms		Extension		
		Flexion		
		Rotation		

WHERE POSSIBLE, ALTERNATE SETS BY CHOOSING TWO VARIATIONS OF EACH EXERCISE

*For an explanation of "supersets," see the description of crunches in Chapter 4.

This basic table provides you with options for creating your own workout program. If you're not the creative type and would like a more programmatic workout schedule, see the back of the book for a six-month schedule based on this table.

THE ART OF CREATING A WORKOUT TAILORED FOR YOUR BODY

Before we get into the details about how to perform each individual exercise, let's talk about some general rules for performing all exercises safely.

RANGE OF MOTION

Most novices concern themselves only with how far they are able to move a weight during a particular exercise. But the distance one can move a weight is not the goal. The goal is to be able to move the weight within a specific, limited range of motion. Exceeding that range of motion, especially with a weight, is never a good idea. Once you exceed the prescribed range of motion, you are no longer targeting the intended muscle. Taking up the stress (that is, bearing the weight) is not the muscle, but the joint structures surrounding the muscle. Such stress can lead to tendonitis or torn ligaments. When your joints are done, you are done.

In the exercise descriptions in the next chapter, therefore, pay particular attention to the range of motion described. Do not lift, pull, push, extend, or rotate beyond the points given.

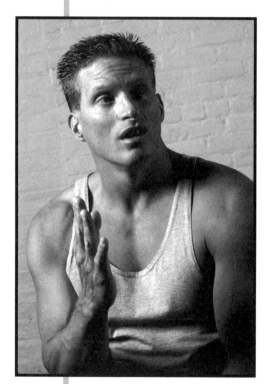

PATH OF MOTION

In addition to staying within each exercise's range of motion, you also want to maintain a safe path of motion throughout the exercise. Think of two sheets of glass running parallel to any working limb or body part. If you don't maintain the correct path of motion in the center of those two sheets of glass — in other words, if your joints are not biomechanically aligned to work most efficiently— then you'd hit the glass and cut yourself.

Maintaining a correct path of motion ensures that the intended muscle is working by contracting. When you do not maintain a correct path of motion, the weight is transferred from your muscles to your joints, subjecting them to undue stress. Muscles lift weight; joints can only bear weight. When you use a joint to bear weight (which will damage the joint in the long run), your body is choosing the path of least resistance—which is not the goal of resistance training. The goal is to isolate a muscle and train it, so that in the course of playing sports and just going about your everyday life, your joints aren't taking all the wear and tear.

If you're moving unintended joints while you're performing an exercise, you're not maintaining your path of motion. Furthermore, if you are either overly rotating a joint that you *are* supposed to use, or otherwise not keeping it in perfect alignment while it's under resistance, you're going to cause damage to that joint.

For example, you may have seen people do dumbbell chest presses and turn their wrists as they get to the top of the movement. That's a huge no-no. Using a joint to bear weight and twisting it at the same time is something your joints were not designed to do.

I was working with a client the other day who's fairly tall and weighs around 250 pounds. He had been trying to lose about 40 pounds, but he complained his workout was giving him shoulder pains. I figured he had impingement problems with his shoulder because he had been pushing too much weight. As I trained him, I showed him how he needed to keep his scapula farther back and down while he lifted the weight. Suddenly, he couldn't lift the 20-pound weight he had been using for months. So I took him down to less than ten pounds, doing the exercise correctly. He said, "Who would ever guess that eight pounds could be so damn heavy?"

I'm also training a woman who's 70 years old. She was in a severe car accident about three years ago and crushed everything on her right leg from her knee down. Since then she's had seven knee operations — after which she couldn't even walk up a flight of stairs. But she comes to the gym religiously and has unbelievable spirit. She said to me the other day, "You have done what all the doctors and physical therapists failed to do—you've given me my life back!" I replied that it wasn't me—all I did was help facilitate the process of her learning to create exercises with her whole body, not just the injured knee. Her rehabilitation was less about the knee and more about her willingness to apply the total-body concepts I was teaching her. This knowledge led her to regain the ability to climb stairs with relative ease—in fact, she climbs no fewer than three flights of stairs before and after each workout we do three times a week.

Another client said to me recently, "I never feel like you're really pushing me, because you don't have to. If I do the exercise the way that you showed me, it just intensifies almost magically, by itself."

I said, "It wasn't magic. Your body has no other recourse *but* to respond in such a dynamic fashion. Therefore, I don't have to push you."

People still have this misconception that they've got to kill themselves or that they need to be sore in order to benefit. You don't have to feel sore to feel like you've used your muscles. Just remember—safety always equals effectiveness and effectiveness always equals safety. The proper form always provides intensity.

MAXIMUM INTENSITY

Here's a technique to increase the intensity of any strength exercise, without even adding weight. It's called "pulsing," and I'll use squats as an example.

First, do ten reps at the full range of motion—squat all the way down, then come all the way back up. Then squat all the way down, hold that position for a couple of seconds, then "pulse" an inch up and an inch back down for ten reps. A pulse is a range of motion of an inch up and an inch back down from the bottom position (or top, in the case of a raising exercise). *Do not bounce*—a pulse is a controlled movement. Pulses intensify the exercise without adding additional resistance. Why? Because you are doing the same amount of work, but in a condensed span of space and time, hence at greater intensity. Greater intensity produces greater results!

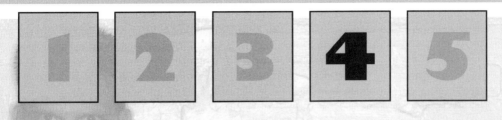

THE
EXTREME WORKOUT

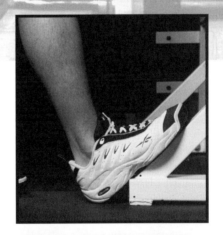

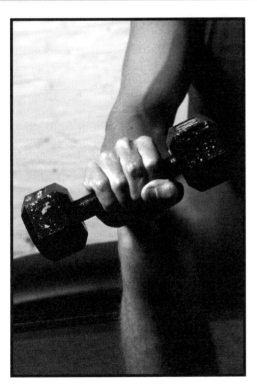

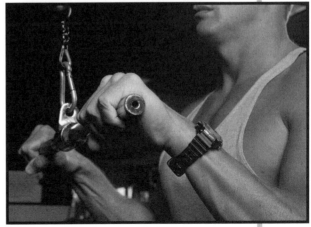

MUSCLE GROUPS	STRETCHES	EXERCISES	LEVEL II (Intermediate)	LEVEL III (Advanced)
LEGS/BUTT:			3–4 sets x 12–15 reps	4 sets x 15–20 reps
Quadriceps	Quad stretch	Athletic squats		
Glutes	Glute stretches (2)	Or: *One-legged squats*		
Abductors/Adductors	Inner thigh stretch	*Ballet squats*		
Hamstrings	Hamstring stretch	*Flexed deadlifts*		
Calves	Calf stretch	*One-leg leg presses*		
		Calf raises		

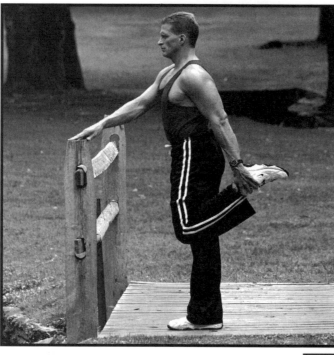

QUAD STRETCH

Grab onto a stationary object with one hand, and grab your opposite ankle with the other hand. Pull up slightly, keeping your thighs parallel to each other. Hold for 15 seconds and switch sides.

In the bad form photo, notice how the thigh is raised up and out.

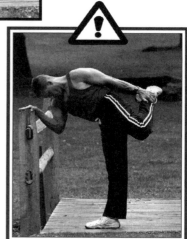

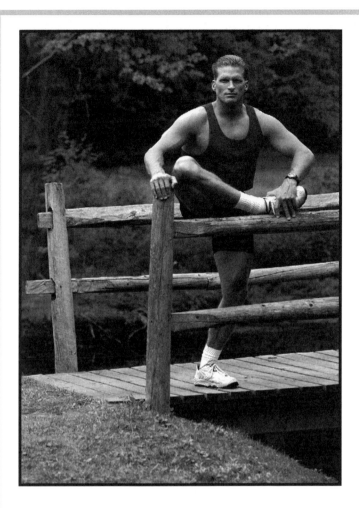

GLUTE STRETCH 1

Place one ankle on a stationary object approximately hip height, as shown. Lean forward slightly. Repeat with the opposite leg.

In the bad form photo, notice how the head and neck are bent over too far.

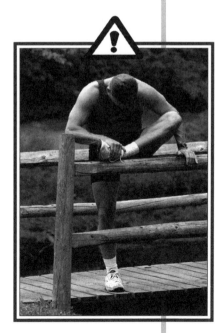

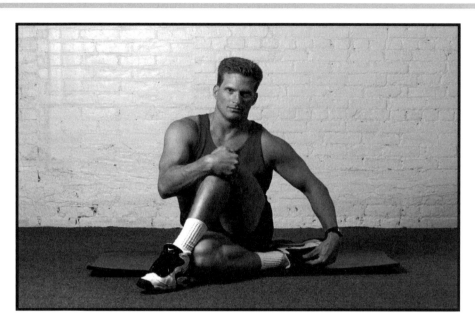

GLUTE STRETCH 2

Sit on the floor with your knees bent and cross one leg over the other, as shown.
Lean in toward your leg. Keep your head up. Repeat with the other leg.

CALF STRETCH

Stand next to an object that
rises off the floor at a 45-
degree angle. Place one foot
along the angle, keeping
your heel on the floor. Center your body weight over
your front ankle. Repeat
with the opposite foot.

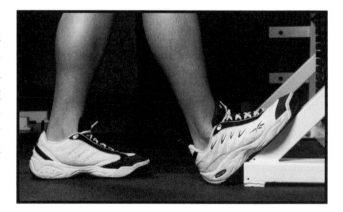

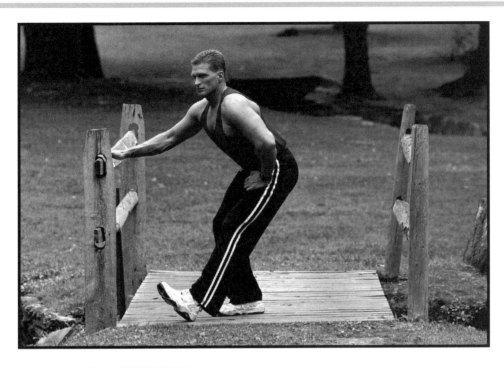

HAMSTRING STRETCH

Grab onto a stable object with one hand. Bend one leg and position the other leg out in front of you as shown. Lean back. Keep the free hand on your thigh. Keep your chest high and your torso upright. Repeat on opposite side.

In the bad form photo, notice how the shoulders are curled in and the head is down.

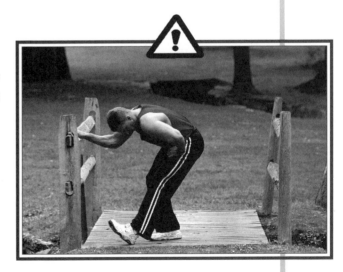

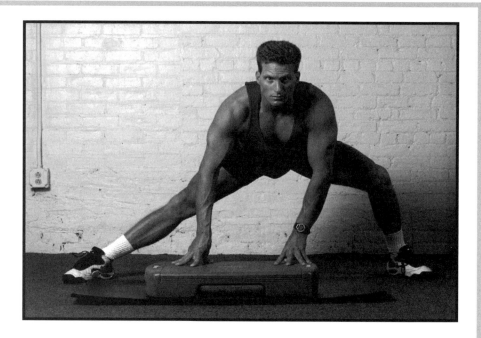

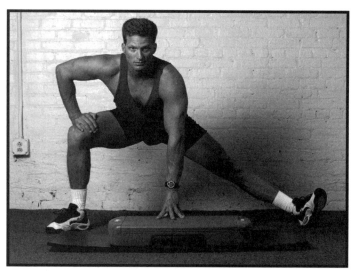

INNER THIGH STRETCH

Lunge to the side with one leg, hold the position for several seconds, then repeat on the opposite side. Both of the forms shown in the photos above are correct; the form in the lower photo is slightly more strenuous (the outstretched leg's heel remains on the floor while the toes point up).

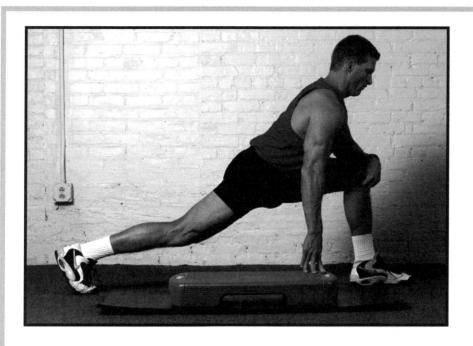

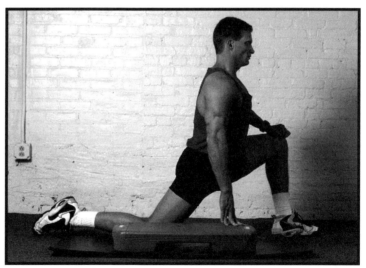

HIP FLEXOR STRETCH

This alternate lower body stretch uses the lunge form to stretch the hip flexors. Repeat stretch on opposite side.

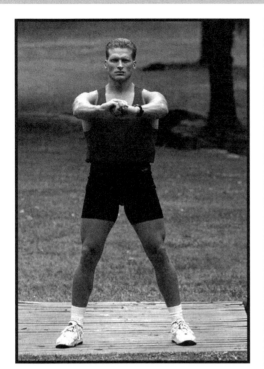
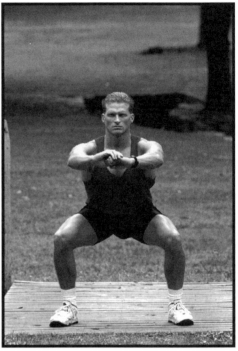
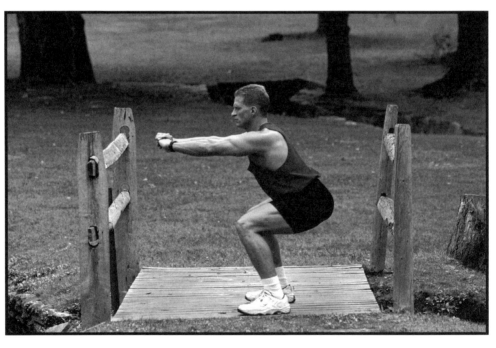

ATHLETIC SQUATS

Stand with your feet shoulder-width apart and your feet slightly turned out. Clasp your hands together out in front of you. As you squat down, do not extend your knees over your toes. Keep your back flat and your head up. Think of sitting back into a chair—squat down directly; don't go forward. You want your thighs to become almost parallel to the ground.

In the bad form photo below, notice how the knees go past the toes, the head is down, and the back is rounded.

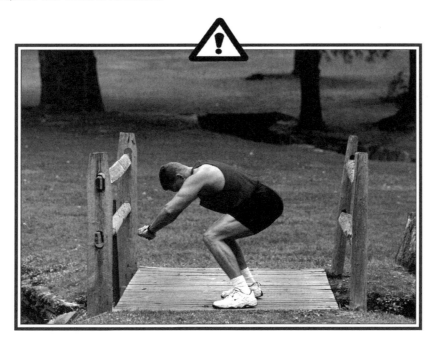

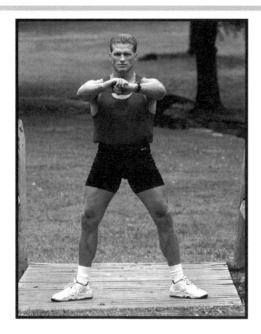
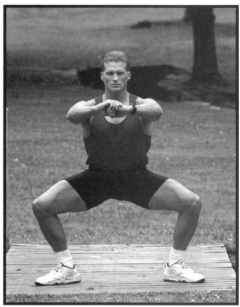

BALLET SQUATS

These squats are similar to athletic squats, only your feet should be further apart and pointed at a 45-degree angle from your torso.

In the bad form photo, note how the torso is pitched forward, putting strain on the knees, which are turned in.

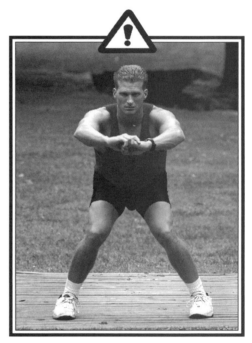

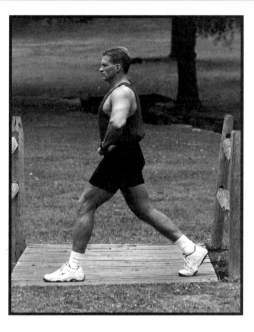 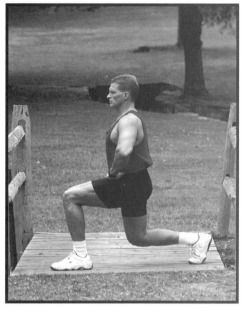

ONE-LEGGED SQUATS

Also known as lunges, in this exercise you want to place your hands on your hips and step forward with one leg. Dip down, keeping your back straight.

Notice how far forward I'm leaning in the bad form photo—keep your back straight and make sure your front knee doesn't go past the front toe.

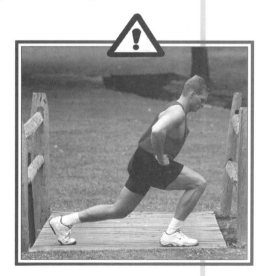

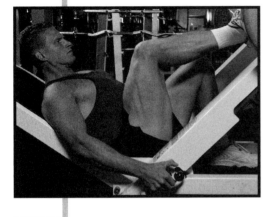

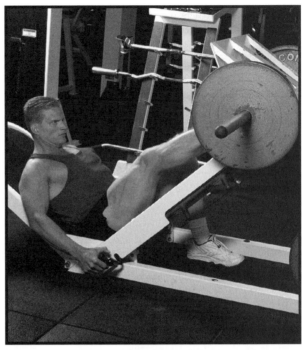

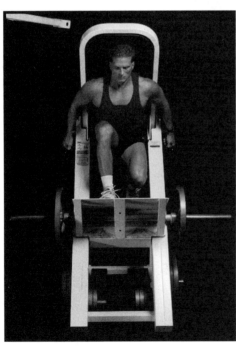

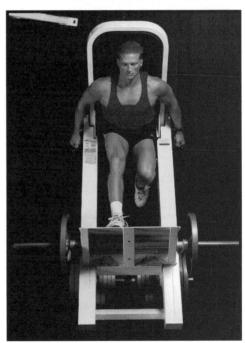

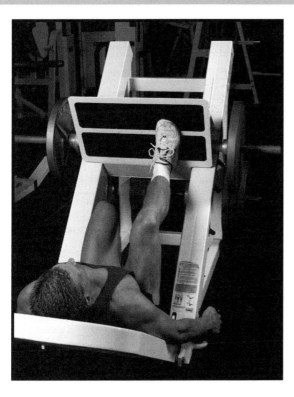

ONE-LEG LEG PRESSES

This is a variation of the standard (two-leg) leg press. Place one foot on the platform where it would be if both your feet were on the platform; in other words, do not "center" your foot on the platform—keep it aligned with your leg. (Notice the poor alignment in the bad form photo.) Start with your leg bent at a 90-degree angle and press until your leg is straight, but your knee is not locked. Maintain continuous tension throughout the movement.

The point of this exercise is to isolate and improve the function of each quadricep; adding more and more weight is not the ultimate goal.

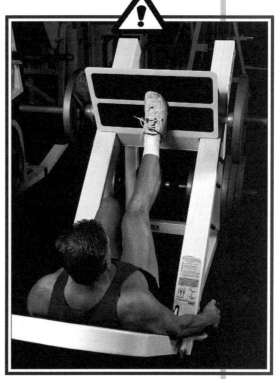

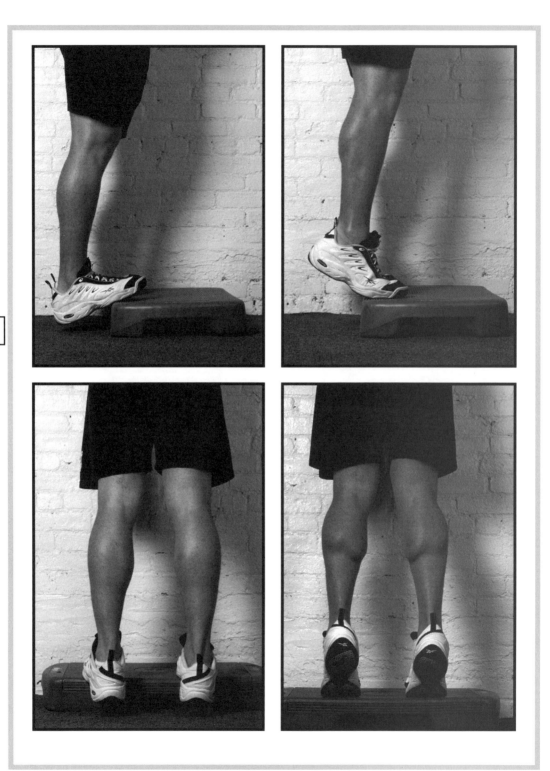

CALF RAISES

With your feet hips-width apart, stand on a step on your toes so that your heels clear the step and your toes are aligned. Drop your heels down, though not excessively (which strains your Achilles tendon). Raise up onto your first and second toes (keep your small toes flat on the step).

In the bad form photo on this page, notice how the toes are pointed outward, rather than straight ahead.

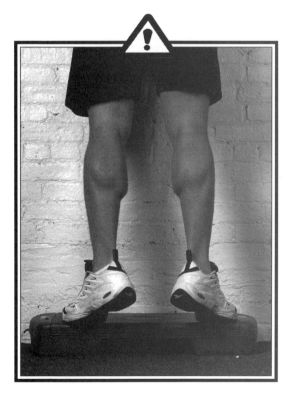

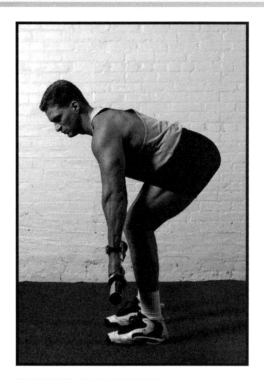
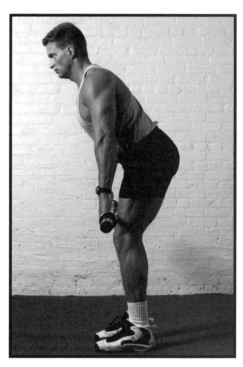

FLEXED DEADLIFTS

Shown here using an easy curl bar, this exercise uses the hamstrings only. Therefore, lift the bar from mid-shin to mid-thigh only (raising it higher engages the glutes). Keep your abs tight and your knees flexed.

In the bad form photo, notice how the back is either excessively arched or rounded and the knees are locked.

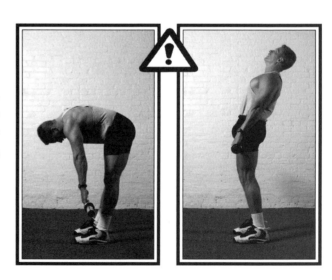

MUSCLE GROUPS	STRETCHES	EXERCISES	LEVEL II (Intermediate)	LEVEL III (Advanced)
ABS AND LOWER BACK:			2–3 supersets* x 20–30 reps	3–4 supersets x 30–50 reps
Abdominals	Knee hug	Basic crunches		
Rectus Abdominus	Back extensions (3)	Advanced crunches		
Obliques	Cat stretch	Reverse crunches		
Erector Spinae				

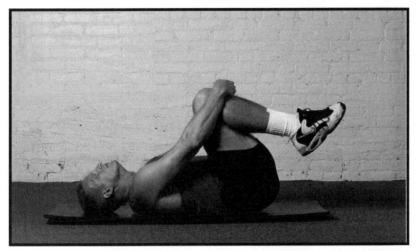

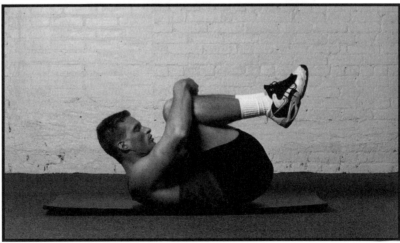

KNEE HUG

This stretch relieves tension in your muscles between sets of crunches. Lie on your back on the floor and put your arms around your knees, as shown. Inhale. Bring your head up to your knees, and hold ten seconds as you exhale.

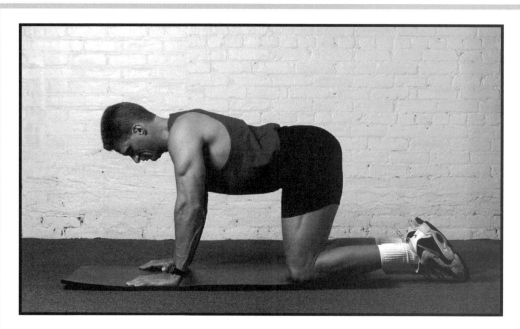

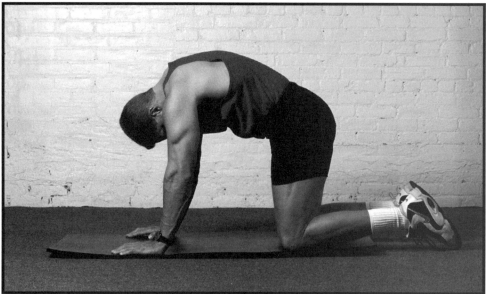

CAT STRETCH

Get down on all fours. Arch your back, pushing your belly toward the floor, then slowly round your back, pulling your belly in.

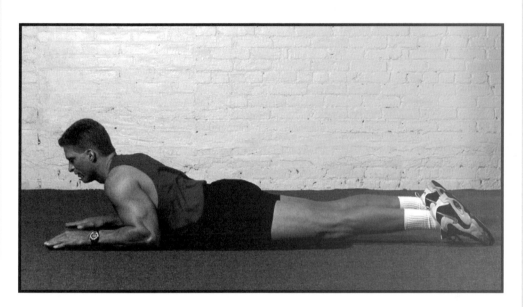

LOWER BACK EXTENSION 1

This stretches your spinal erectors. Lie on your stomach and raise up on your upper arms, keeping your palms face down and your elbows tucked next to your body. Your chest should come off the floor, but do not raise up any higher.

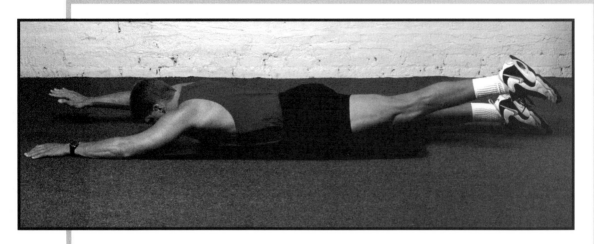

LOWER BACK EXTENSION 2

Lie on your stomach with your hands outstretched over your head. Keeping your head down, lift one arm and the opposite leg two or three inches off the ground for three to five seconds. Repeat with the opposite limbs. Then, raise both arms and legs off the floor simultaneously. (This position is also known as the "super-man.")

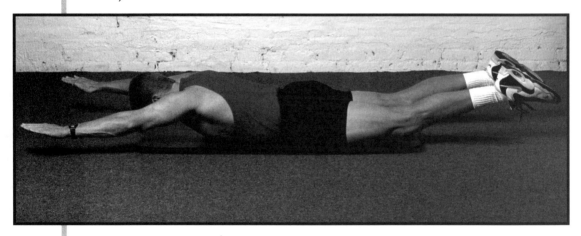

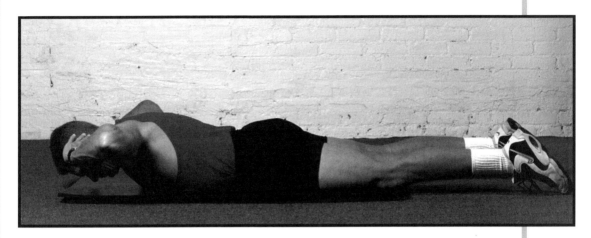

LOWER BACK EXTENSION 3

Lie on your stomach with your hands behind your head, as shown. Raise your chest off the floor. You won't be able to come very high off the floor; don't force the stretch.

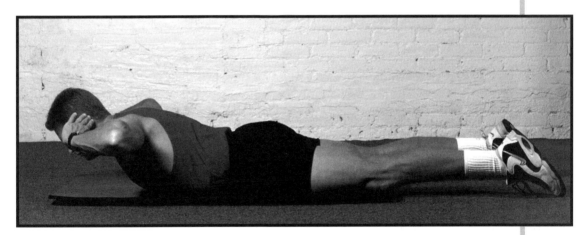

AB SUPERSETS

The most common abdominal exercises are crunches. People often confuse crunches with their popular predecessor, sit-ups. What's the difference between a sit-up and a crunch? In a crunch, after you lift your shoulder blades off the ground, you do not lower them all the way back down again until you've completed all your reps.

Although the range of motion in a crunch is much smaller than in a sit-up, crunches are much more difficult. You may be able to do hundreds of sit-ups, but only a few crunches! (As fitness professionals like to say about any exercise, if you do 'em wrong, you can do 'em all day long.)

The idea behind crunches is to maintain continuous tension in the abdominal muscles. Doing so makes crunches much more effective than sit-ups—and that's what it's all about.

Furthermore, by limiting the range of motion, crunches are easier on your back than sit-ups. Think of a credit card that you bend slightly in one direction. What if you started bending it in the opposite direction—forward and back, forward and back? It would snap! Well, you don't want to do that to your back, do you?

As you're doing the following crunches, think of sliding your sternum toward your pelvis, rather than lifting your chest off the ground.

In the following descriptions, we'll take you through four variations of the crunch, each one more difficult than the last. When you can complete two sets of 20 to 30 reps of each crunch easily, taking a rest of less than 30 seconds between sets (don't worry—it may take a while!), do one ab "superset": 20 to 30 reps of each type of crunch with *no* rest between variations. When you need to challenge yourself even more, try to do two to three supersets.

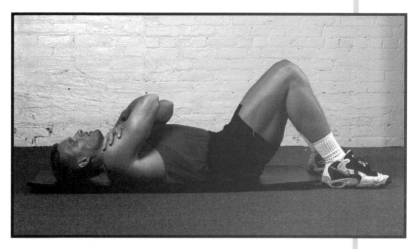

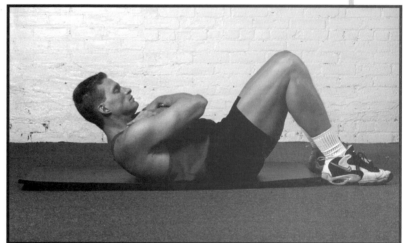

BASIC CRUNCHES

Lie on your back with your knees bent up and your feet flat on the floor. Cross your hands over your chest. Do *not* interlock your hands behind your head—you can pull on your neck and cause injury. Crunch up, bringing your head toward your knees and slowly lowering it again—but not all the way to the floor! Keep your shoulder blades just off the floor. Do not crane up—think of sliding toward your pelvis and shortening the distance between it volves a very small range of motion.

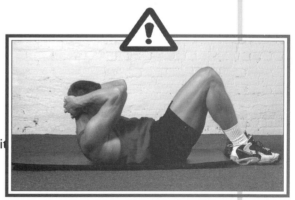

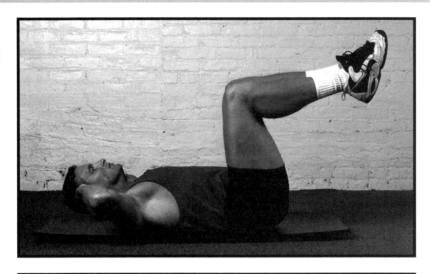

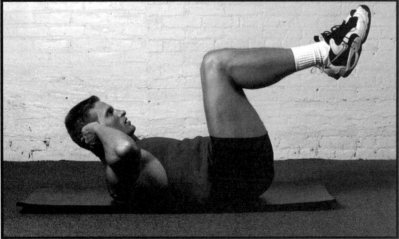

ADVANCED CRUNCHES

Assume the same starting position as the basic crunch, only bring your feet off the ground, so that your shins form a 90-degree angle with your thighs. Place your hands at your ears and lift your head off the ground. This is the starting position. Slide your chest toward your knees while keeping your feet off the ground and your legs level. Do *not* cross your ankles—doing so can pull your lower back.

For an even more advanced crunch, bring your knees toward your chest while you bring your chest toward your knees.

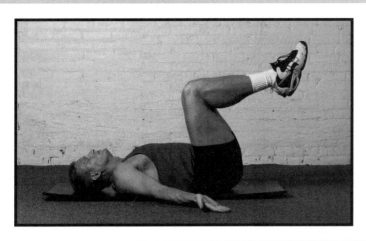

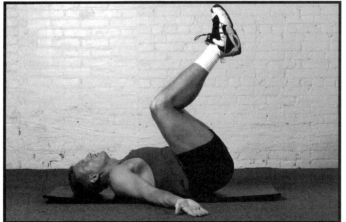

REVERSE CRUNCHES

Assume the same position as the advanced crunch, only place your arms flat at your sides with your palms up (this discourages you from using your arms for leverage). Raise your pelvis and lower again. Think about rolling your hips toward your sternum, not up toward the sky. You want to keep the movement on a horizontal plane. This crunch works the lower portion of your abdominal muscles.

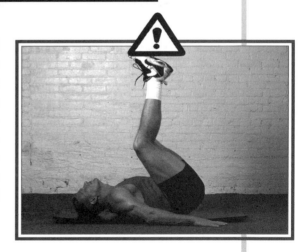

MUSCLE GROUPS	STRETCHES	EXERCISES	LEVEL II (Intermediate)	LEVEL III (Advanced)
CHEST:			3–4 sets x 10–12 reps	4 sets x 8–10 reps
Pectoralis Major	Standing pec stretch	Push-ups		
		Or: Incline bench presses		
		Dumbbell presses		
		Bench push-ups		
		Standing cable flyes		

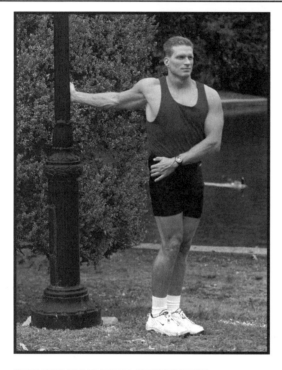

STANDING PEC STRETCH

Grab a secure object at shoulder height with one hand. With your arm outstretched, slightly turn away from the arm (do not turn excessively). Hold the stretch for 15 seconds and repeat on other side.

Do not turn your shoulder in, bend your neck down, or hold the object too high, as shown in the bad form photo.

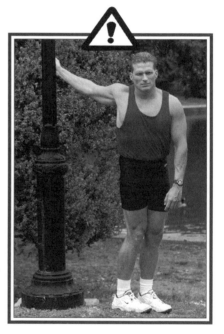

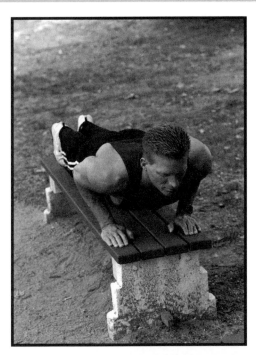

PUSH-UPS

You can do these from your knees with your feet in the air or from your toes. In either case, place your hands shoulder-width apart. Make sure you look forward, not down, as you do the push-ups. Keep your abs tight, your back flat (not swayed), and your head up. While push-ups mainly work the chest muscles, they also work the triceps and abs.

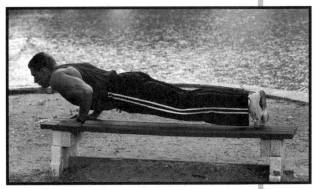

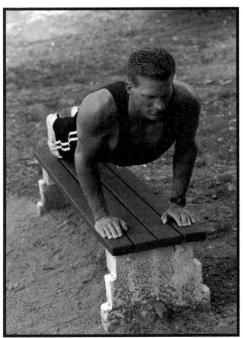

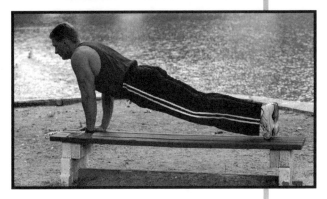

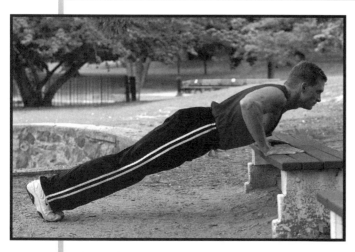

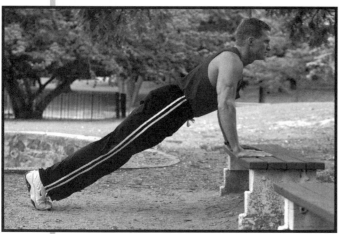

BENCH PUSH-UPS

Doing push-ups on an incline changes the resistance on your pectoral muscles. When you do a push-up with your feet elevated on a bench, you must push greater resistance (your raised legs), thereby making this alternative harder. Remember to keep your back flat.

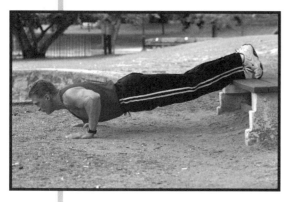

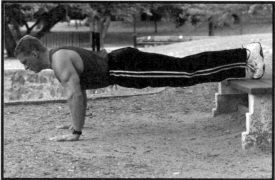

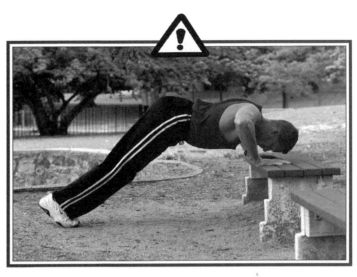

In these bad form photos, note how the butt is elevated, breaking the body's alignment, and the head is down.

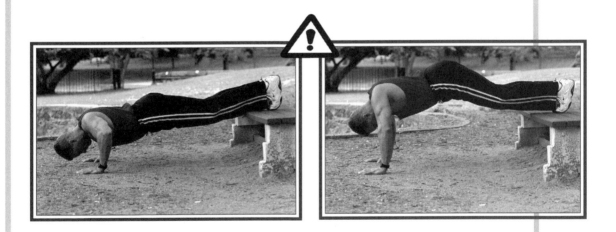

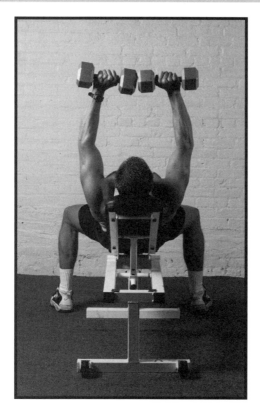 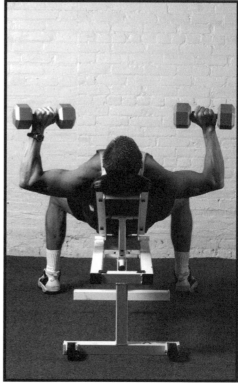

INCLINE BENCH PRESSES

Incline the bench to no higher than 35 degrees (any higher forces you to engage your deltoids). Grasp dumbbells in each hand with your palms facing away from you. To start, hold the dumbbells in fully extended arms over the mid-line of your chest. Depress your scapula, pressing your shoulder blades into the back of the bench. Bring the dumbbells down, bending your elbows. Do not drop your elbows below your body at the bottom, which stresses the shoulder joints, and do not lock your elbows at the top, as shown in the bad form photos on the next page.

By inclining the bench, you are changing the angle of resistance and forcing the pectoral muscles to adapt to a stress that is slightly different from a flat bench press or a push-up.

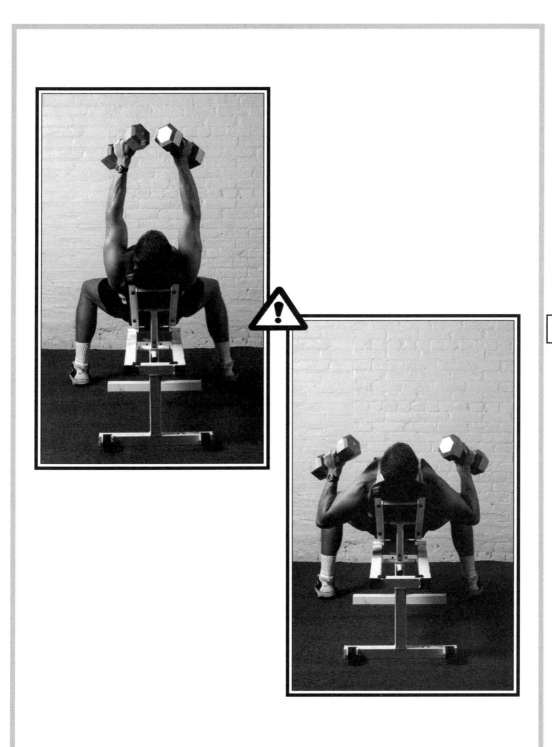

THE EXTREME WORKOUT

STANDING CABLE FLYES

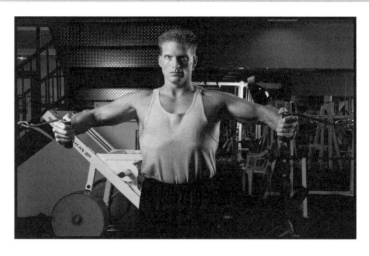

You must use an adjustable cross-cable machine for this exercise. Adjust the cables so that they cross the mid-section of your chest. Start with a 90-degree angle at your elbows, which should be slightly in front of your body. Keep a slight flex in your elbows throughout the movement. Do not drop your elbows down; keep them parallel to the floor. Note how, in the last photo below, my grip is different. By starting and finishing the exercise with your palms facing down, you can turn the exercise into a cable press. Never switch your grip (turn your palms) while executing the exercise, though!

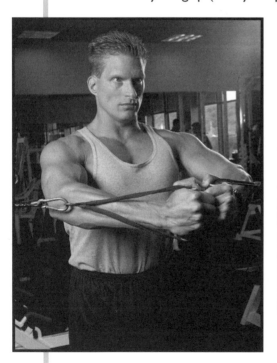

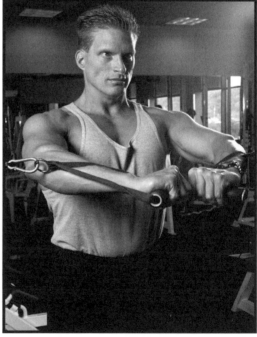

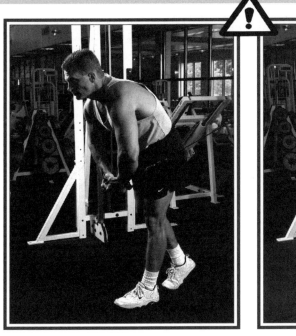
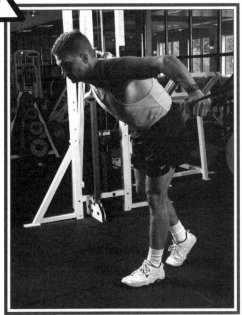

In the bad form photos, notice how I am leaning forward (a big no-no) and pulling the cables to below waist level rather than to chest level. In the last photo, notice how my elbows are not bent at 90-degree angles to start.

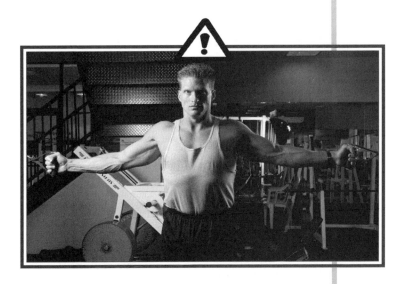

MUSCLE GROUPS	STRETCHES	EXERCISES	LEVEL II (Intermediate)	LEVEL III (Advanced)
UPPER BACK:			3–4 sets x 12–15 reps	4 sets x 8–10 reps
Latissimus Dorsi	Lat stretch	Pull-ups		
		Single-arm dumbbell rows		
		Or: *Reverse-grip pull-downs*		
		Straight-arm lat pull-downs		

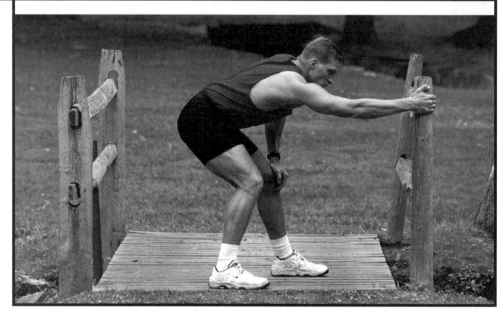

LAT STRETCH

With your knees slightly bent and your back flat, grab a stationary object with one arm and lean back. Feel the stretch in your back. Hold for 15 seconds and repeat on other side.

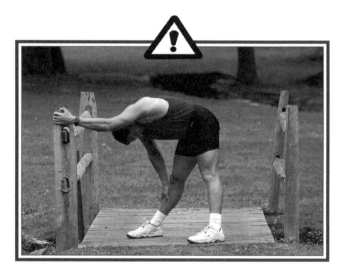

In the bad form photo, notice how the head is down and the knees are locked.

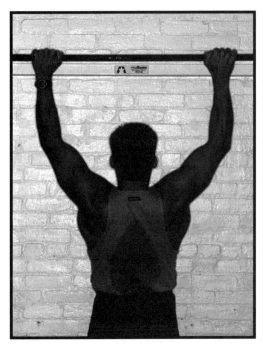

PULL-UPS

Your grip on the bar should be over-hand and slightly wider than shoulder width. Pull your chin up to the bar.

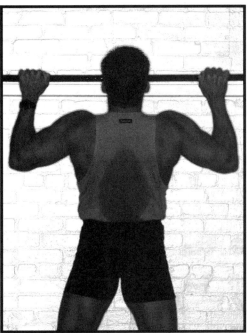

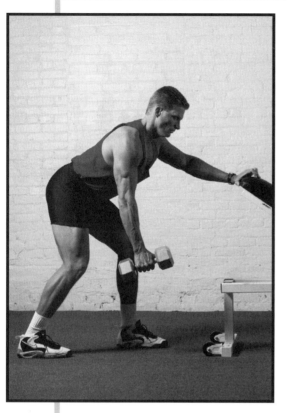

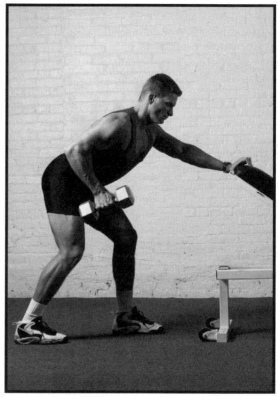

SINGLE-ARM DUMBBELL ROWS

Hold a dumbbell in one arm, place the opposite arm on a stationary object, and step forward with one foot, as shown. Your weight should be evenly distributed among your legs and your supportive arm. Bring the dumbbell up toward your hip (do not bring it up all the way to your armpits, as in the bad form photo). Keep your back flat and your head up.

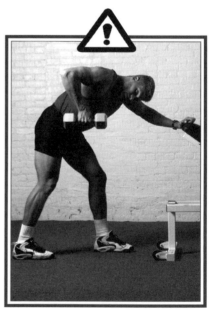

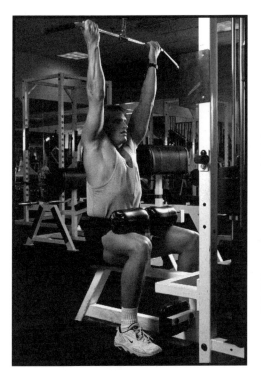
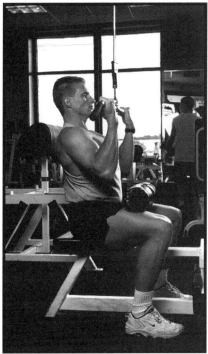

REVERSE-GRIP PULL-DOWNS

Sit with the pad above your thighs. You should hold the bar with a slightly wider than shoulder-width undergrip. Make sure your back is straight and your abs are tight. Depress your scapula, then pull the bar to chin level. Do *not* pull down or press down behind your head—this can cause injury to your shoulder. Unfortunately, this is a very common mistake. Also, do not lean back and pull to your chest—as in the bad form photo—doing so uses your biceps, which is not the aim of this exercise.

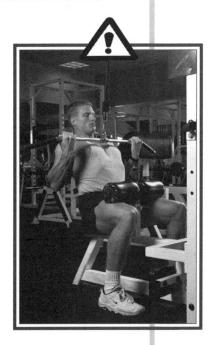

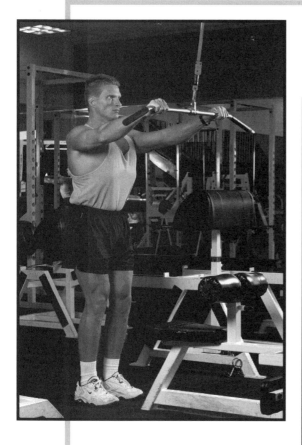

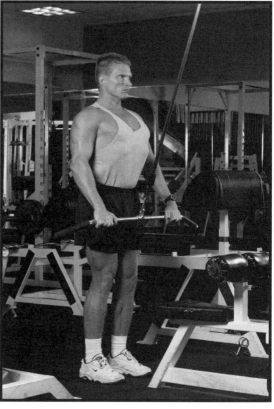

STRAIGHT-ARM LAT PULL-DOWNS

Stand with your back straight, abs tight, and shoulder blades retracted. Your arms should be straight, with a slight flex in your elbow throughout the motion. To start, the bar should be at eye level. Think of squeezing your lats while you bring the bar down to thigh level. Keep your back sturdy.

In the bad form photos, notice how I'm starting with the bar too high, finishing with the bar too low, and leaning in. These mistakes are very common.

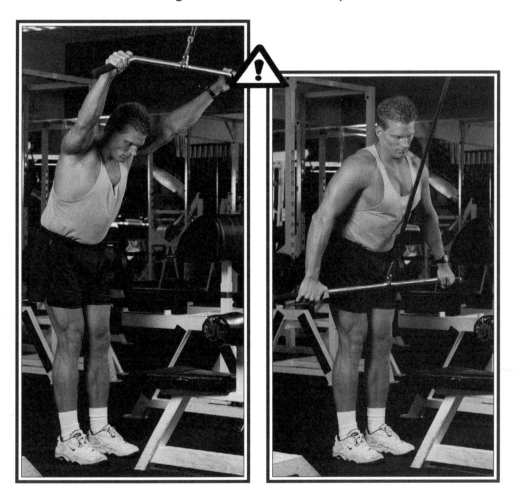

MUSCLE GROUPS	STRETCHES	EXERCISES	LEVEL II (Intermediate)	LEVEL III (Advanced)
SHOULDERS AND UPPER BACK:			3 sets x 12–15 reps	4 sets x 10–12 reps
Deltoids	Shoulder stretch	Barbell clean-presses		
Trapezius	Neck stretch	Or: Seated dumbbell presses		
		Dumbbell lateral raises		
		Or: Bent-over rear delt raises		

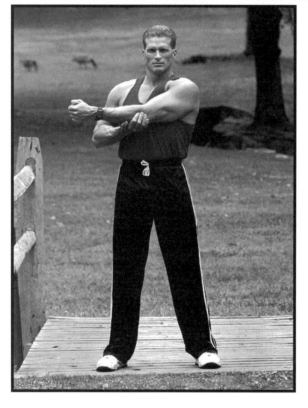

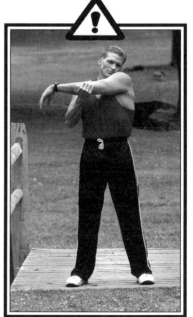

SHOULDER STRETCH

Hold one bent elbow with your opposite hand and slightly pull it across your body. Keep your shoulder relaxed. Hold for 15 seconds and repeat on opposite side.

Note, in the bad form photo, how the neck is tilted and the arm is pulled higher.

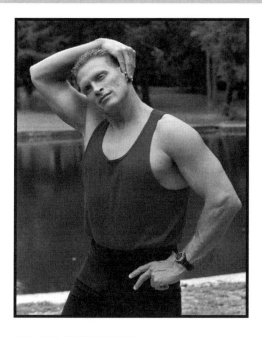
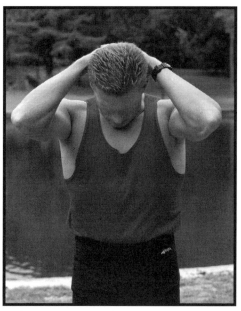

NECK STRETCH

Place one hand on the opposite side of your head, and tilt your head to the side, as shown. Repeat on the opposite side. Then put both hands on the back of your head and bring your chin toward your chest. Do not tilt your head back—doing so can damage the cartilage in your neck.

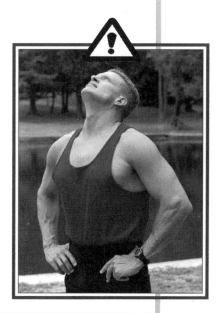

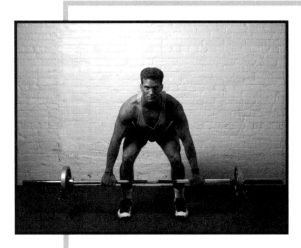

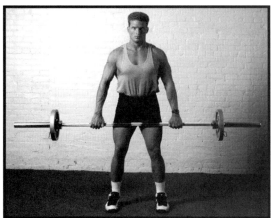

BARBELL CLEAN-PRESSES

This advanced exercise is a total body exercise, as you raise the barbell from the floor to your chin. During the entire exercise, keep your knees flexed, your abs tight, your head up, and your back straight. Using a slightly wider than shoulder-width grip, raise the barbell from the floor up to your hips in a standing position, then up to your chin. In the same controlled movement, return the barbell to the floor.

If you have a bad back, you can raise the barbell off a power rack at thigh level, rather than off the floor.

A common mistake with this exercise is trying to lift too much weight. Don't be overzealous!

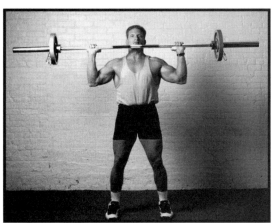

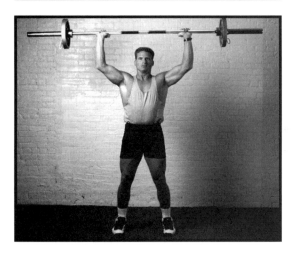

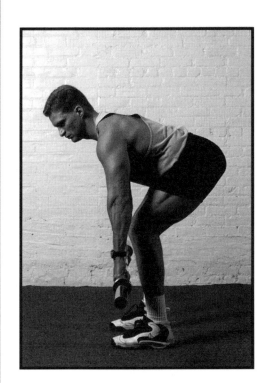

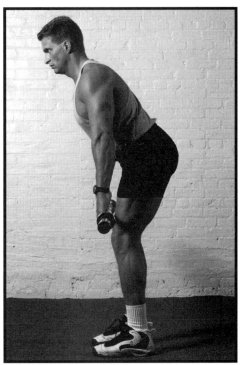

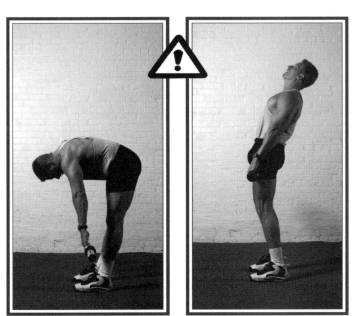

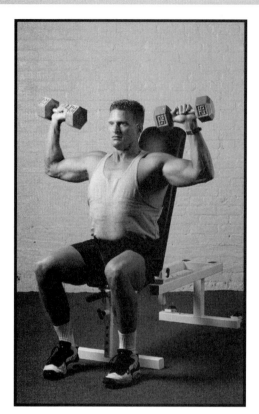
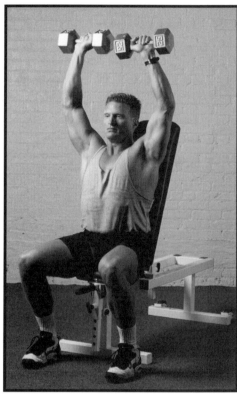

SEATED OVERHEAD DUMBBELL PRESSES

Sit on the bench with your feet flat on the floor. The bench doesn't need to be completely vertical, but it should support your lower back. Hold the dumbbells out to your sides at ear level and depress your scapula. Raise the dumbbells overhead, being careful not to lock your elbows at the top. Keep the space between your ears and elbows as open as possible. This exercise works your deltoids.

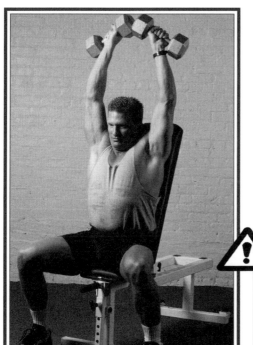

Be sure to keep your elbows and hands completely vertical to avoid putting undue pressure on your joints (see bad form photo at right).

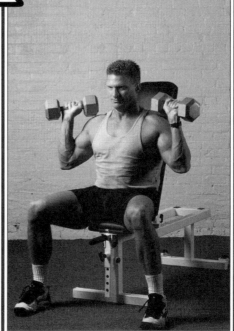

THE EXTREME WORKOUT

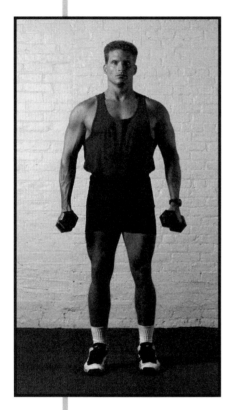

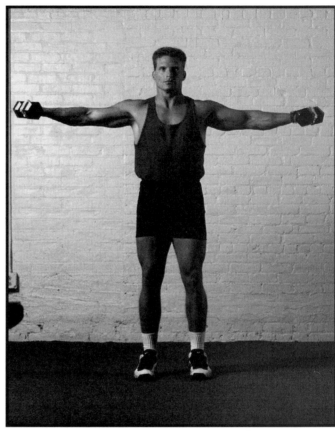

DUMBBELL LATERAL RAISES

This is the most common incorrectly performed exercise. Stand straight with your feet shoulder-width apart and knees slightly flexed. Hold the dumbbells in your hands with your palms facing down, elbows slightly bent, and arms at your sides. Raise your arms slowly up to the shoulders, exhaling as you do so. Hold for two counts and slowly return to starting position, inhaling slowly. Keep a slight bend in your elbow throughout the entire range of motion. Do not raise the dumbbells over your shoulders, which will place stress on the shoulders and may injure the rotator cuff. Concentrate on extending your arms laterally before lifting them straight up.

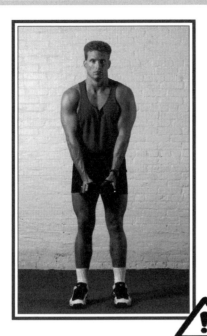

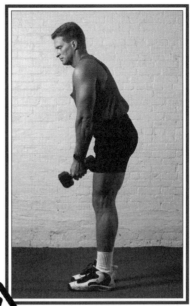

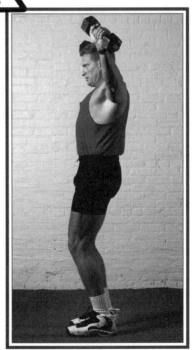

In bad form, people often use momentum, throwing their arms up and back, which can hurt their shoulders. In the bad form photos, notice how the dumbbells are in front of my body at the start, I raise them too high at the top, and my elbows are excessively bent.

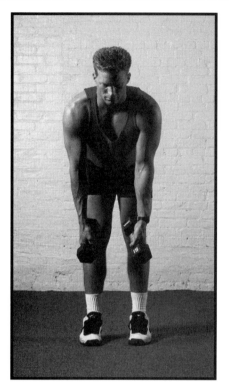

BENT-OVER REAR DELT RAISES

Bend over, keeping your back flat, your abs tight, and a slight bend in your knees. Retract your shoulder blades and hold the dumbbells at shin level. Raise your elbows out and up—do not swing them back. Use a modest weight when performing this exercise, as it targets only one aspect of the deltoids.

A common mistake with this exercise is to use momentum to "swing" your arms up and back. Doing so can injure your shoulders.

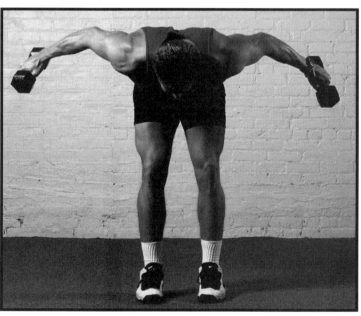

MUSCLE GROUPS	STRETCHES	EXERCISES	LEVEL II (Intermediate)	LEVEL III (Advanced)
ARMS (FRONT):			3 sets x 12–15 reps	3–4 sets x 10–12 reps
Biceps	Bicep stretch	Standing barbell curls		
		Alternating dumbbell curls		
		Or: *Hammer curls*		
		Cable bicep curls		

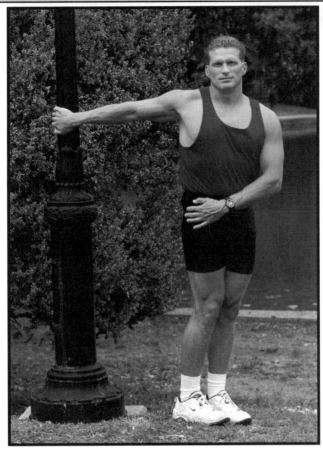

BICEP STRETCH

This is the same form as the pec stretch on page 64, only the grip is reversed so that the thumb points down. Grab a secure object with one hand. With your arm outstretched, slightly turn away from the arm (do not turn excessively). Hold the stretch for 15 seconds and repeat on other side.

Do not turn your shoulder in, bend your neck down, or hold the object too high.

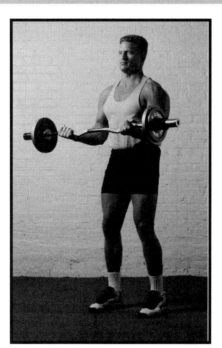 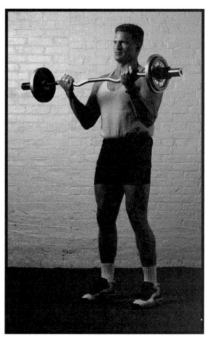

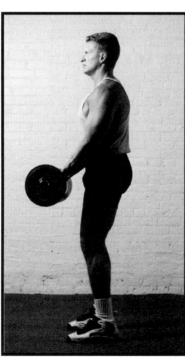 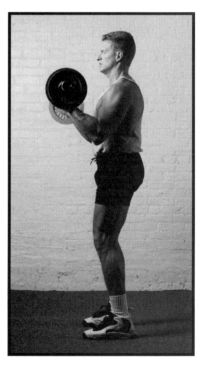

EXTREME TRAINING

STANDING BARBELL CURLS

Stand straight with your feet shoulder-width apart. Hold the barbell in front of you with a slightly wider than shoulder-width underhand grip. Lift bar to shoulder level and slowly lower down again. Do not curl your wrist.

Notice how the back is arched in the bad form photos below.

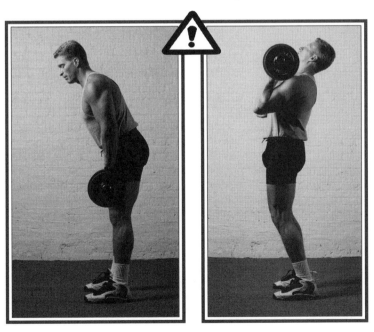

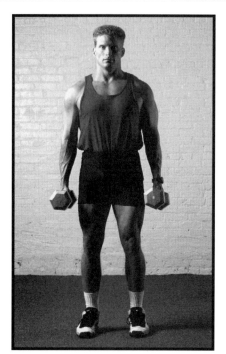
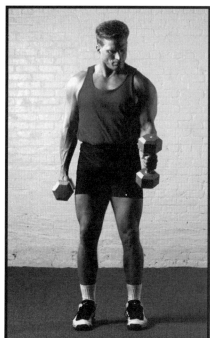
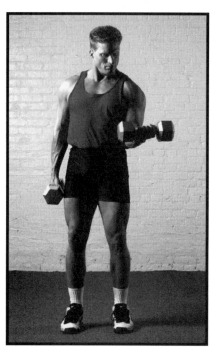
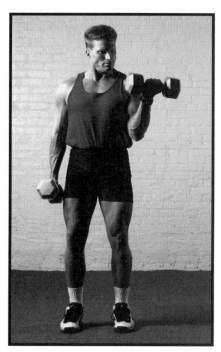

ALTERNATING DUMBBELL CURLS

Stand, holding dumbbells in each hand at your sides so that your palms face your legs. Raise one dumbbell at a time to your chest: Pull one dumbbell forward (using your forearm muscle), and as the dumbbell clears your thigh, turn your wrist so that your palm faces your body, using your bicep to raise the dumbbell to your chest. Turn your wrist back again on its way down. Perform this exercise in a slow and controlled motion. Do not switch arms until the one arm has completed the motion.

Be careful not to lean your back to the side, as shown in the bad form photo.

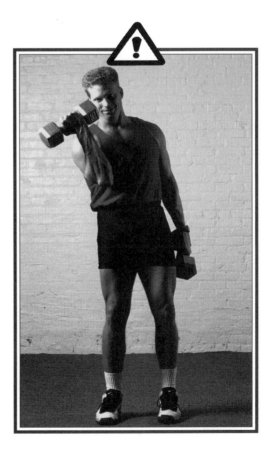

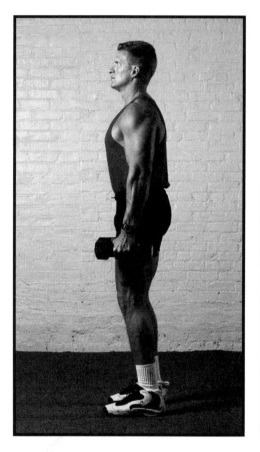 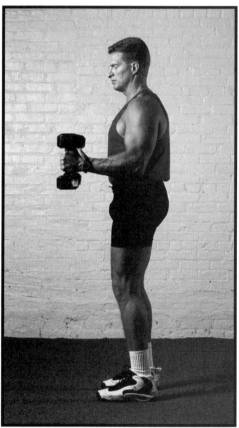

HAMMER CURLS

Begin in the same starting position as alternating dumbbell curls, holding the dumbbells in the "hammer" position (as you would hold a hammer, with your palms facing toward your body). Raise the dumbbells only high enough for a 90-degree angle to form at your elbows, while maintaining the hammer-like grip.

MUSCLE GROUPS	STRETCHES	EXERCISES	LEVEL II (Intermediate)	LEVEL III (Advanced)
ARMS (BACK):			3 sets x 12–15 reps	3–4 sets x 10–12 reps
Triceps	Tricep stretch	Bench dips		
		Overhead dumbbell extensions		
		Or: *Dumbbell kickbacks*		
		Cable tricep extensions		
Forearms		Extension		
		Flexion		

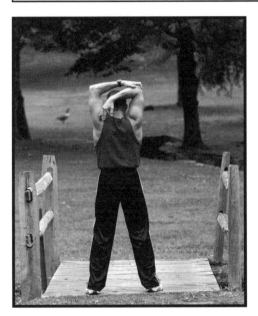

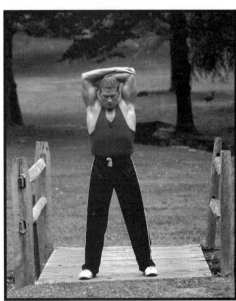

TRICEP STRETCH

Grab one elbow behind your head with the opposite hand. Do not yank your body to the side. Hold and repeat on the opposite side.

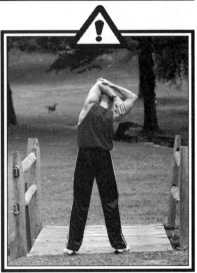

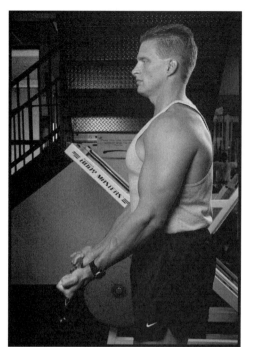

CABLE BICEP CURLS

Keeping a slight bend in your knees, your back straight, and your abs tight, stand close to and parallel to the cable, with your elbows slightly in front of your body, not cocked in back of your body. Your hands should be shoulder-width apart on the bar. As you curl the cable up, keep your wrists straight, not curled back. Concentrate on maintaining continuous tension in your biceps. The only moving joints should be the elbows; keep the rest of your body motionless. Raise the cable only to shoulder level, not chin level.

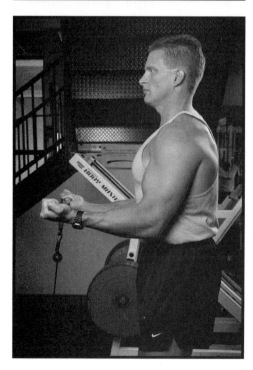

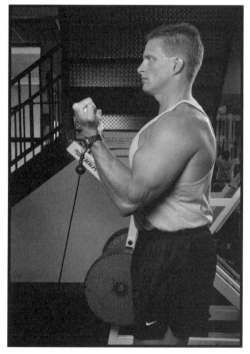

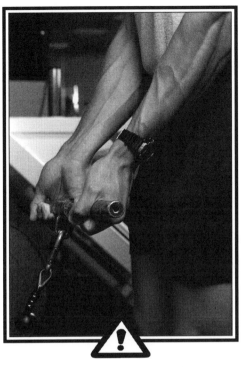

Note how my hands are too close together in the bad form photo above. Below, I'm leaning forward, pulling the cable too close to my body, pulling the cable too high, and leaning back—all bad form!

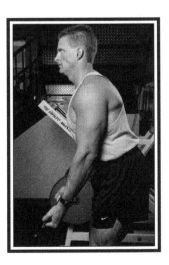
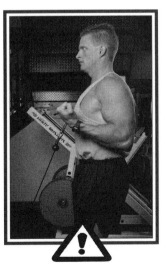
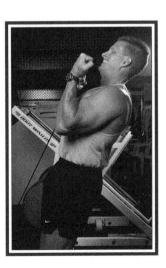

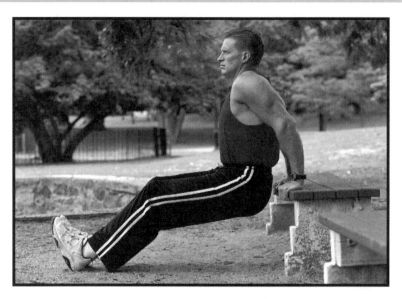

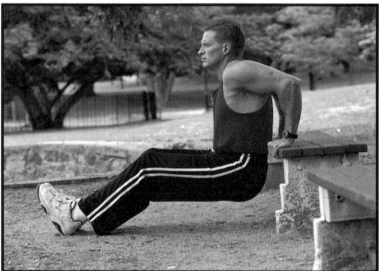

BENCH DIPS

Sit on a bench with your knees bent at 90-degree angles. Move your torso forward, balancing your upper body on your arms on the bench. Rest your legs on your heels. Dip your butt straight down toward the ground, then raise back up. Do not dip too far down, past the 90-degree angle that is formed at your elbows.

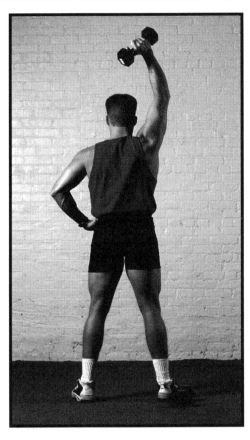
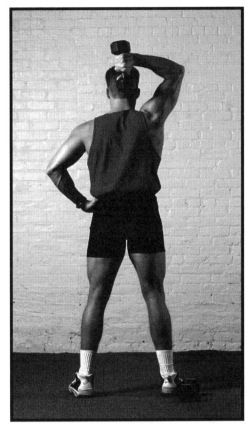

OVERHEAD DUMBBELL EXTENSIONS

Stand with your knees slightly bent, your abs tight, back straight, scapula depressed, and one hand on your hip. With a dumbbell in the other hand, fully extend that arm over your head. Bend your elbow, bringing the dumbbell back behind your head. Keep your wrist straight. Repeat with the opposite arm.

In the bad form photos, the dumbbell starts too far out to the side and then is brought too far down the back.

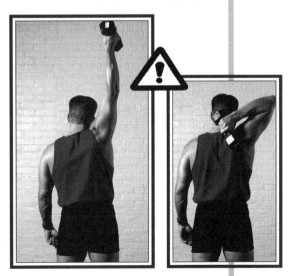

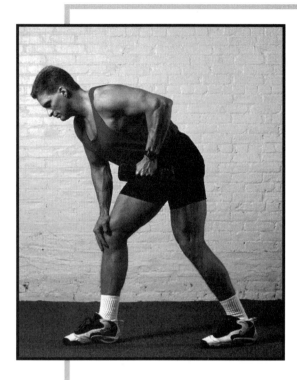

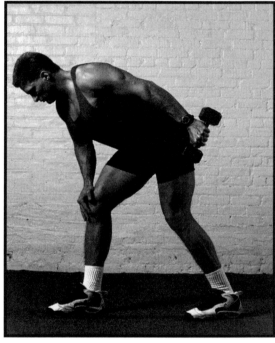

DUMBBELL KICKBACKS

Step forward and put one hand on the forward knee to support your upper body. Hold a dumbbell in the other hand at your waist, then extend your arm straight back. *Do not swing* your arm back. Repeat with the other arm. This exercise is the same as the overhead dumbbell extension; your body has just changed position.

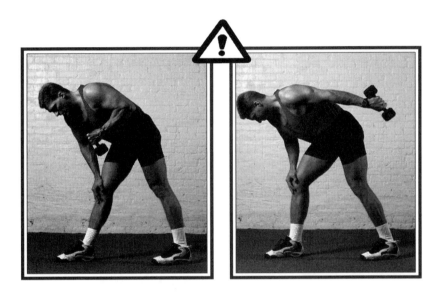

In the bad form photos, the dumbbell is held at the chin to start and swung back too high.

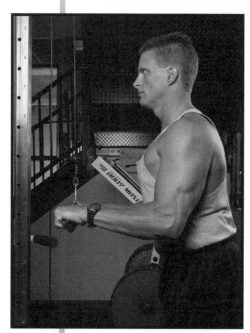

CABLE TRICEP EXTENSIONS

To start, your elbows should be bent at 90-degree angles. Press the cables down to thigh level. Keep your elbows straight, but do not force the lock. Push out, then down. If your body is moving up and down, you're not using your triceps. No wrist action is involved.

For variation, you can use either grip shown in the two close-up photos. (The different grips have no particular advantages or disadvantages.)

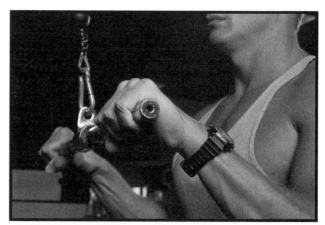

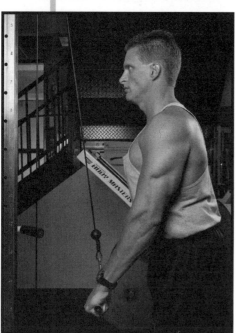

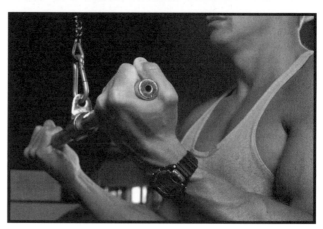

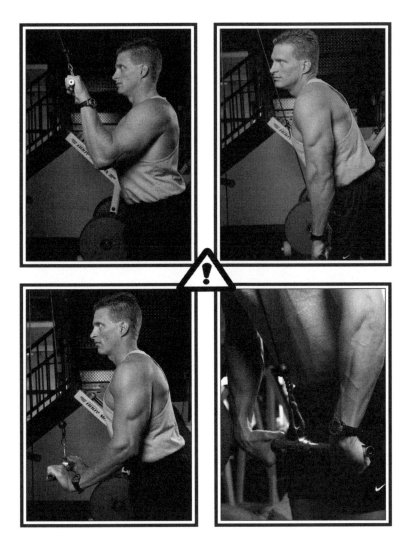

These bad form photos show a starting position that is too high, a finishing position too low, and bad wrist form.

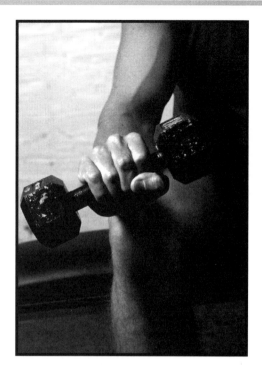 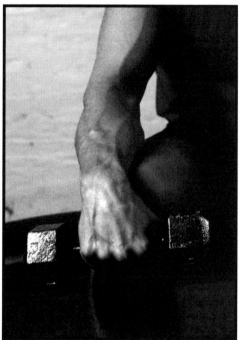

FOREARM EXTENSION

For the next three forearm exercises, which involve very small muscles, use a very light weight. These exercises help improve your grip strength. (Bear in mind, however, in most sports, the common mistake is to "overgrip" or "overtense" your muscles when holding, say, a golf club or a tennis racquet—doing so is a waste of energy and can hurt your game.)

While sitting, rest your forearms on your thighs so that your wrists clear your knees. Hold dumbbells in your hands (within your fingertips), with your palms facing down. Slowly curl your wrists up.

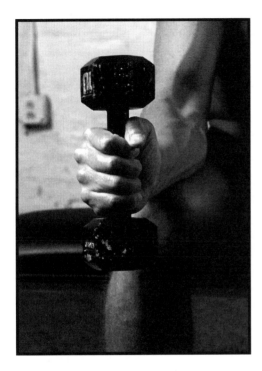 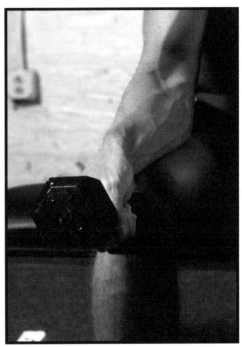

FOREARM FLEXION

In the same position as forearm extension, hold the dumbbells in the hammer position and raise and lower them.

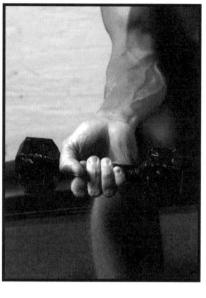
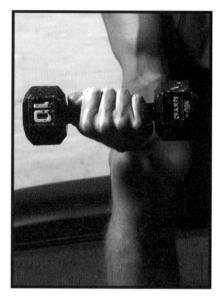

FOREARM ROTATION

In the same basic position, hold the dumbbells so that your palms are facing up, then slowly rotate your wrists over so that your palms are facing down.

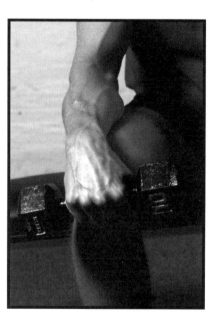
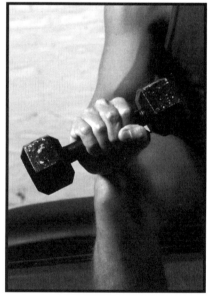

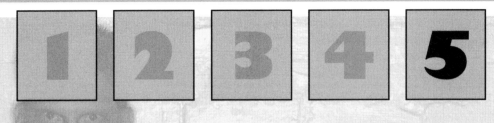

THE MIND: THE KEY TO UNLOCKING YOUR INDIVIDUAL PHYSICAL POTENTIAL

WHAT SEPARATES OLYMPIC ATHLETES from the rest of us? Genetic good fortune? Perhaps, in some cases. Sponsorship that allows them to train—or be massaged—for hours on end? Perhaps, to some degree. But the most important factor separating them from other mere mortals is this: their mental discipline.

So much for "dumb jocks"! World-class athletes must have amazing powers of concentration. During performance, they visualize in their minds the moves they want to execute in order to prepare their muscles. During training, they concentrate on what each exercise is trying to accomplish. How does this make their training and performance more effective?

For one thing, it keeps them motivated. I look around the gym and see women reading the newspaper on the treadmill and guys doing dumbbell curls with their eyes glazed over. These people are not thinking about what they're doing. There's no mental aspect to their workout. If your mind is wandering during your workout, you're definitely going to fall into a rut.

The truth is, most people don't achieve their fitness goals because of mental weakness. They don't suffer from genetic disadvantages or from a lack of desire. It's a lack of concentration they suffer from.

As you do the exercises as they're described in Chapter 4, mentally talk yourself through them. Which muscle are you (and should you) be working?

Many fitness pros have catchy names for exercises, but you'll notice that I name exercises by the muscles they're working. This helps remind me what muscle, exactly, I'm training. By thinking about the muscle while you're working it, you'll be able to tell how much stronger it feels since the last time you did the exercise. You'll be better able to judge when it's appropriate to add reps, add weight, or try a different exercise altogether.

It's been said that your flesh and bones are your body's hardware and your mind is the software. It doesn't matter how good the hardware is if the software isn't running!

VISUALIZATION

The first mental challenge you face is to have a realistic image of yourself today and a realistic image of what you can look like with exercise. Unfortunately, we are surrounded by ads in glossy magazines that are all designed to get our attention and convey the message: "This *can* be you (if you just buy…)!" These images trade in misinformation and have power in people's minds. Shaking their influence takes concentration.

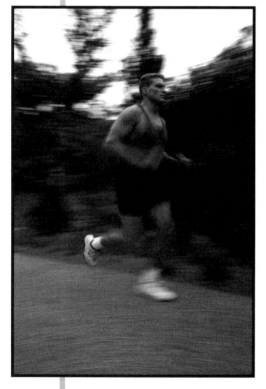

You can't help but notice ads that promise, "Immediate results after your first visit to our gym!" You may want more than anything to believe that. But you know better, especially after reading the first few chapters about what exactly exercise can and cannot do for you.

Why do you think tanning salons are still so popular? After all, everyone knows tanning is very bad for the skin. It's because tanning salons deliver the holy grail of advertising: immediate results. It's the ultimate example of buy now, pay later.

So how do you block out all these unrealistic images? With the constant bombardment of ads, information, and retouched images, we live in a distracted society. How is anyone able to concentrate on anything—and block out everything else?

Thinking, believe it or not, takes practice. It takes discipline to keep all those unrealistic images and desires in your subconscious from breaking into your conscious efforts. Typically, when I'm halfway through training a client on his or her first day, the client says to me, "There's a lot more to this than I thought there was!" I'm not having them do any more exercises than any other trainer—I'm just having them *think* more about what they're doing.

Concentration, however, doesn't mean *overthinking*. Relax. Don't get uptight or you will be tempted to push yourself too hard. Let your body do its job. Realize that, once

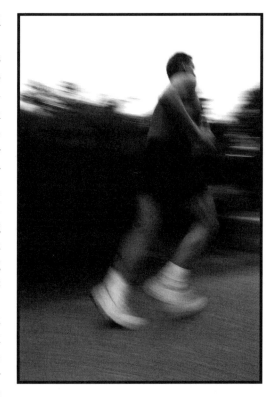

you start exercising correctly, nothing you do or take is going to speed up the process. Your desire alone is not going to change your physiology, and you can waste a lot of energy trying to look like some guy in an ad for a nutritional supplement. If you harbor false beliefs, you're going to defeat yourself mentally before you even begin.

TRAIN YOUR MIND

You've got to train your mind, just as you train your muscles. Do mini-mental workouts: Take five or ten minutes a couple times a day, when you're *not* exercising, and mentally rehearse your workout. Go through each exercise you plan to do during your workout, telling yourself why and how you're going to do it. Think about the benefits that each exercise will bring. Think about performing the exercise correctly, in the proper range of motion, and maintaining the proper path of motion.

You may think doing "mental workouts" sounds silly. But don't you mentally rehearse important situations all the time? Like how you're going to ask the boss for a raise, how you're going to ask that pretty girl out on a date, how you're going to beat Michael Jordan if you two should ever get into a game of one-on-one…. It's human nature to visualize events before we execute them. And there's sound physiological evidence to suggest that mental "rehearsals" have physical benefits—that there is a mind-muscle link.

For instance, the *Newsweek* article "Music on the Mind" (July 24, 2000) examined the effects of physical vs. mental practice among people being taught to play piano:

Researchers led by Dr. Alvaro Pascual-Leone of Beth Israel taught nonmusicians a simple five-finger piano exercise. The volunteers practiced in the lab two hours a day for five days. Not surprisingly, the amount of territory the brain devotes to moving the fingers expanded. But then the scientists had another group think only about practicing—that is, the volunteers mentally rehearsed the five-finger sequence, also for two hours at a time. "This changed the cortical map just the way practicing physically did," says Pascual-Leone. "They make fewer mistakes when they played, just as few mistakes as people actually practicing for five days. *Mental and physical practice improves performance more than physical practice alone, something we can now explain physiologically.*" [ital. added]

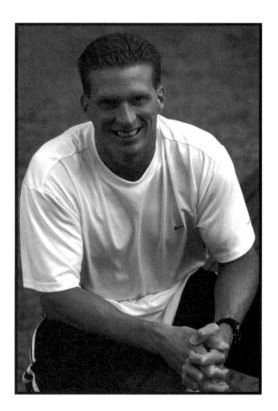

Physical ability alone won't get you there. You need mental discipline. Block out life's stresses and distractions. Give yourself pep talks. Be your own trainer. You have all the knowledge you need now to design your own workout program and, most important, realize your own individual physical potential.

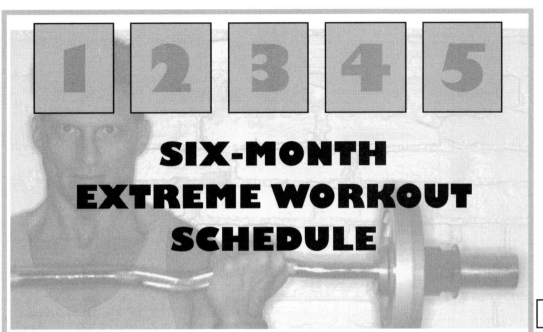

SIX-MONTH EXTREME WORKOUT SCHEDULE

THE WORKOUT TABLE PRESENTED IN CHAPTER 4 gives you all the various exercises you can do to work each muscle group. From that table, you can design your own workout, based on your fitness level, which exercises give you the best results, and which exercises you enjoy. Some exercises involve gym equipment; others you can do at home or outside. The table offers a Chinese menu of exercise options.

The key to an effective workout is to mix up the exercises—don't always do athletic squats, for example. After a couple weeks, do the one-leg leg press instead. In this way, you keep your body challenged without necessarily adding more weight or reps right away.

If creativity is not your strong suit, this appendix presents a six-month (26-week) workout that is based on the workout table presented in Chapter 3. Do each strength-training workout three times a week for two weeks. (Remember: Do not strength train two days in row, and leave one a day a week for no training whatsoever.) In addition, make sure you get in your 30 minutes of cardio training three times a week. It is a good idea to change your cardio workout every two weeks as well: Go from jogging to biking to interval training of each, for example. The stretches are not included in the following tables, but do remember to stretch (1) after you've warmed up, (2) in between sets of strength training exercises, or (3) after your workout.

STRENGTH TRAINING WORKOUT: 3 TIMES A WEEK

❏ ❏ ❏	Athletic squats	3 sets of 12 to 15 reps
❏ ❏ ❏	Calf raises	3 sets of 12 to 15 reps
❏ ❏ ❏	Basic crunches	2 supersets* of 20 to 30 reps
❏ ❏ ❏	Advanced crunches	2 supersets of 20 to 30 reps
❏ ❏ ❏	Reverse crunches	2 supersets of 20 to 30 reps
❏ ❏ ❏	Push-ups	3 sets of 10 to 12 reps
❏ ❏ ❏	Pull-ups	3 sets of 12 to 15 reps
❏ ❏ ❏	Single-arm dumbbell rows	3 sets of 12 to 15 reps
❏ ❏ ❏	Barbell clean-presses	3 sets of 12 to 15 reps
❏ ❏ ❏	Dumbbell lateral raises	3 sets of 12 to 15 reps
❏ ❏ ❏	Standing barbell curls	3 sets of 12 to 15 reps
❏ ❏ ❏	Alternating dumbbell curls	3 sets of 12 to 15 reps
❏ ❏ ❏	Bench dips	3 sets of 12 to 15 reps
❏ ❏ ❏	Overhead dumbbell extensions	3 sets of 12 to 15 reps
❏ ❏ ❏	Forearm extension	3 sets of 12 to 15 reps
❏ ❏ ❏	Forearm flexion	3 sets of 12 to 15 reps
❏ ❏ ❏	Forearm rotation	3 sets of 12 to 15 reps

* See Chapter 4 for an explanation of "supersets."

CARDIO TRAINING WORKOUT: 30 MINUTES, 3 TIMES A WEEK

Type of cardio activity: _____

Interval training? ❏ Yes   ❏ No

STRETCHES: INCORPORATE INTO EACH DAY'S WORKOUT

- Quad stretch
- Glute stretches
- Inner thigh stretch
- Hamstring stretch
- Calf stretch
- Knee hug
- Back extensions
- Cat stretch
- Standing pec stretch
- Lat stretch
- Shoulder stretch
- Neck stretch
- Bicep stretch
- Tricep stretch

STRENGTH TRAINING WORKOUT: 3 TIMES A WEEK

☐ ☐ ☐ One-legged squats .... 3 sets of 12 to 15 reps
☐ ☐ ☐ Calf raises.. 3 sets of 12 to 15 reps
☐ ☐ ☐ Basic crunches .... 2 supersets of 20 to 30 reps
☐ ☐ ☐ Advanced crunches .... 2 supersets of 20 to 30 reps
☐ ☐ ☐ Reverse crunches .... 2 supersets of 20 to 30 reps
☐ ☐ ☐ Incline bench presses .... 3 sets of 10 to 12 reps
☐ ☐ ☐ Reverse-grip pulldowns .... 3 sets of 12 to 15 reps
☐ ☐ ☐ Straight-arm lat pulldowns .... 3 sets of 12 to 15 reps
☐ ☐ ☐ Seated dumbbell presses .... 3 sets of 12 to 15 reps
☐ ☐ ☐ Bent-over rear delt raises .... 3 sets of 12 to 15 reps
☐ ☐ ☐ Hammer curls .... 3 sets of 12 to 15 reps
☐ ☐ ☐ Cable bicep curls .... 3 sets of 12 to 15 reps
☐ ☐ ☐ Dumbbell kickbacks .... 3 sets of 12 to 15 reps
☐ ☐ ☐ Cable tricep extensions .... 3 sets of 12 to 15 reps
☐ ☐ ☐ Forearm extension .... 3 sets of 12 to 15 reps
☐ ☐ ☐ Forearm flexion .... 3 sets of 12 to 15 reps
☐ ☐ ☐ Forearm rotation .... 3 sets of 12 to 15 reps

CARDIO TRAINING WORKOUT: 30 MINUTES, 3 TIMES A WEEK

Type of cardio activity: _____

Interval training? ☐ Yes   ☐ No

STRETCHES: INCORPORATE INTO EACH DAY'S WORKOUT

- Quad stretch
- Glute stretches
- Inner thigh stretch
- Hamstring stretch
- Calf stretch
- Knee hug
- Back extensions
- Cat stretch
- Standing pec stretch
- Lat stretch
- Shoulder stretch
- Neck stretch
- Bicep stretch
- Tricep stretch

III

STRENGTH TRAINING WORKOUT: 3 TIMES A WEEK

❑ ❑ ❑ Ballet squats .... 4 sets of 12 to 15 reps
❑ ❑ ❑ Calf raises .... 4 sets of 12 to 15 reps
❑ ❑ ❑ Basic crunches .... 3 supersets of 20 to 30 reps
❑ ❑ ❑ Advanced crunches .... 3 supersets of 20 to 30 reps
❑ ❑ ❑ Reverse crunches .... 3 supersets of 20 to 30 reps
❑ ❑ ❑ Dumbell presses .... 4 sets of 10 to 12 reps
❑ ❑ ❑ Pull-ups .... 4 sets of 12 to 15 reps
❑ ❑ ❑ Reverse-grip pulldowns .... 4 sets of 12 to 15 reps
❑ ❑ ❑ Barbell clean presses .... 3 sets of 12 to 15 reps
❑ ❑ ❑ Bent-over rear delt raises .... 3 sets of 12 to 15 reps
❑ ❑ ❑ Standing barbell curls .... 3 sets of 12 to 15 reps
❑ ❑ ❑ Cable bicep curls .... 3 sets of 12 to 15 reps
❑ ❑ ❑ Bench dips .... 3 sets of 12 to 15 reps
❑ ❑ ❑ Cable tricep extensions .... 3 sets of 12 to 15 reps
❑ ❑ ❑ Forearm extension .... 3 sets of 12 to 15 reps
❑ ❑ ❑ Forearm flexion .... 3 sets of 12 to 15 reps
❑ ❑ ❑ Forearm rotation .... 3 sets of 12 to 15 reps

CARDIO TRAINING WORKOUT: 30 MINUTES, 3 TIMES A WEEK

Type of cardio activity: _____

Interval training? ❑ Yes ❑ No

STRETCHES: INCORPORATE INTO EACH DAY'S WORKOUT

- Quad stretch
- Glute stretches
- Inner thigh stretch
- Hamstring stretch
- Calf stretch
- Knee hug
- Back extensions
- Cat stretch
- Standing pec stretch
- Lat stretch
- Shoulder stretch
- Neck stretch
- Bicep stretch
- Tricep stretch

STRENGTH TRAINING WORKOUT: 3 TIMES A WEEK

☐ ☐ ☐ Flexed deadlifts .... 4 sets of 12 to 15 reps
☐ ☐ ☐ Calf raises .... 4 sets of 12 to 15 reps
☐ ☐ ☐ Basic crunches .... 3 supersets of 20 to 30 reps
☐ ☐ ☐ Advanced crunches .... 3 supersets of 20 to 30 reps
☐ ☐ ☐ Reverse crunches .... 3 supersets of 20 to 30 reps
☐ ☐ ☐ Bench push-ups .... 4 sets of 10 to 12 reps
☐ ☐ ☐ Single-arm dumbbell rows .... 4 sets of 12 to 15 reps
☐ ☐ ☐ Straight-arm lat pulldowns .... 4 sets of 12 to 15 reps
☐ ☐ ☐ Seated dumbbell presses .... 3 sets of 12 to 15 reps
☐ ☐ ☐ Dumbbell lateral raises .... 3 sets of 12 to 15 reps
☐ ☐ ☐ Standing barbell curls .... 3 sets of 12 to 15 reps
☐ ☐ ☐ Hammer curls .... 3 sets of 12 to 15 reps
☐ ☐ ☐ Overhead dumbbell extensions .... 3 sets of 12 to 15 reps
☐ ☐ ☐ Cable tricep extensions .... 3 sets of 12 to 15 reps
☐ ☐ ☐ Forearm extension .... 3 sets of 12 to 15 reps
☐ ☐ ☐ Forearm flexion .... 3 sets of 12 to 15 reps
☐ ☐ ☐ Forearm rotation .... 3 sets of 12 to 15 reps

113

CARDIO TRAINING WORKOUT: 30 MINUTES, 3 TIMES A WEEK

Type of cardio activity: _____

Interval training? ☐ Yes ☐ No

STRETCHES: INCORPORATE INTO EACH DAY'S WORKOUT

- Quad stretch
- Glute stretches
- Inner thigh stretch
- Hamstring stretch
- Calf stretch
- Knee hug
- Back extensions
- Cat stretch
- Standing pec stretch
- Lat stretch
- Shoulder stretch
- Neck stretch
- Bicep stretch
- Tricep stretch

STRENGTH TRAINING WORKOUT: 3 TIMES A WEEK

❑ ❑ ❑ One-leg leg presses .... 4 sets of 12 to 15 reps
❑ ❑ ❑ Calf raises .... 4 sets of 12 to 15 reps
❑ ❑ ❑ Basic crunches .... 3 supersets of 20 to 30 reps
❑ ❑ ❑ Advanced crunches .... 3 supersets of 20 to 30 reps
❑ ❑ ❑ Reverse crunches .... 3 supersets of 20 to 30 reps
❑ ❑ ❑ Standing cable flyes .... 4 sets of 10 to 12 reps
❑ ❑ ❑ Reverse-grip pulldowns .... 4 sets of 12 to 15 reps
❑ ❑ ❑ Straight-arm lat pulldowns .... 4 sets of 12 to 15 reps
❑ ❑ ❑ Seated dumbbell presses .... 3 sets of 12 to 15 reps
❑ ❑ ❑ Bent-over rear delt raises .... 3 sets of 12 to 15 reps
❑ ❑ ❑ Cable bicep curls .... 3 sets of 12 to 15 reps
❑ ❑ ❑ Hammer curls .... 3 sets of 12 to 15 reps
❑ ❑ ❑ Overhead dumbbell extensions .... 3 sets of 12 to 15 reps
❑ ❑ ❑ Bench dips .... 3 sets of 12 to 15 reps
❑ ❑ ❑ Forearm extension .... 3 sets of 12 to 15 reps
❑ ❑ ❑ Forearm flexion .... 3 sets of 12 to 15 reps
❑ ❑ ❑ Forearm rotation .... 3 sets of 12 to 15 reps

CARDIO TRAINING WORKOUT: 30 MINUTES, 3 TIMES A WEEK

Type of cardio activity: _____

Interval training? ❑ Yes   ❑ No

STRETCHES: INCORPORATE INTO EACH DAY'S WORKOUT

- Quad stretch
- Glute stretches
- Inner thigh stretch
- Hamstring stretch
- Calf stretch
- Knee hug
- Back extensions
- Cat stretch
- Standing pec stretch
- Lat stretch
- Shoulder stretch
- Neck stretch
- Bicep stretch
- Tricep stretch

114

STRENGTH TRAINING WORKOUT: 3 TIMES A WEEK

☐ ☐ ☐ Athletic squats .... 4 sets of 15 to 20 reps
☐ ☐ ☐ Calf raises .... 4 sets of 15 to 20 reps
☐ ☐ ☐ Basic crunches .... 3 supersets of 30 to 50 reps
☐ ☐ ☐ Advanced crunches .... 3 supersets of 30 to 50 reps
☐ ☐ ☐ Reverse crunches .... 3 supersets of 30 to 50 reps
☐ ☐ ☐ Push-ups .... 4 sets of 8 to 10 reps
☐ ☐ ☐ Pull-ups .... 4 sets of 8 to 10 reps
☐ ☐ ☐ Single-arm dumbbell rows .... 4 sets of 8 to 10 reps
☐ ☐ ☐ Barbell clean-presses .... 4 sets of 10 to 12 reps
☐ ☐ ☐ Dumbbell lateral raises .... 4 sets of 10 to 12 reps
☐ ☐ ☐ Standing barbell curls .... 3 sets of 10 to 12 reps
☐ ☐ ☐ Alternating dumbbell curls .... 3 sets of 10 to 12 reps
☐ ☐ ☐ Bench dips .... 3 sets of 10 to 12 reps
☐ ☐ ☐ Overhead dumbbell extensions .... 3 sets of 10 to 12 reps
☐ ☐ ☐ Forearm extension .... 3 sets of 10 reps
☐ ☐ ☐ Forearm flexion .... 3 sets of 10 reps
☐ ☐ ☐ Forearm rotation .... 3 sets of 10 reps

CARDIO TRAINING WORKOUT: 30 MINUTES, 3 TIMES A WEEK

Type of cardio activity: _____

Interval training? ☐ Yes ☐ No

STRETCHES: INCORPORATE INTO EACH DAY'S WORKOUT

• Quad stretch
• Glute stretches
• Inner thigh stretch
• Hamstring stretch
• Calf stretch
• Knee hug
• Back extensions
• Cat stretch
• Standing pec stretch
• Lat stretch
• Shoulder stretch
• Neck stretch
• Bicep stretch
• Tricep stretch

115

STRENGTH TRAINING WORKOUT: 3 TIMES A WEEK

❏ ❏ ❏ One-legged squats .... 4 sets of 15 to 20 reps
❏ ❏ ❏ Calf raises .... 4 sets of 15 to 20 reps
❏ ❏ ❏ Basic crunches .... 3 supersets of 30 to 50 reps
❏ ❏ ❏ Advanced crunches .... 3 supersets of 30 to 50 reps
❏ ❏ ❏ Reverse crunches .... 3 supersets of 30 to 50 reps
❏ ❏ ❏ Incline bench presses .... 4 sets of 8 to 10 reps
❏ ❏ ❏ Reverse-grip pulldowns .... 4 sets of 8 to 10 reps
❏ ❏ ❏ Straight-arm lat pulldowns .... 4 sets of 8 to 10 reps
❏ ❏ ❏ Seated dumbbell presses .... 3 sets of 10 to 12 reps
❏ ❏ ❏ Bent-over rear delt raises .... 3 sets of 10 to 12 reps
❏ ❏ ❏ Hammer curls .... 3 sets of 10 to 12 reps
❏ ❏ ❏ Cable bicep curls .... 3 sets of 10 to 12 reps
❏ ❏ ❏ Dumbbell kickbacks .... 3 sets of 10 to 12 reps
❏ ❏ ❏ Cable tricep extensions .... 3 sets of 10 to 12 reps
❏ ❏ ❏ Forearm extension .... 3 sets of 10 reps
❏ ❏ ❏ Forearm flexion .... 3 sets of 10 reps
❏ ❏ ❏ Forearm rotation .... 3 sets of 10 reps

CARDIO TRAINING WORKOUT: 30 MINUTES, 3 TIMES A WEEK

Type of cardio activity: _____

Interval training? ❏ Yes   ❏ No

STRETCHES: INCORPORATE INTO EACH DAY'S WORKOUT

- Quad stretch
- Glute stretches
- Inner thigh stretch
- Hamstring stretch
- Calf stretch
- Knee hug
- Back extensions
- Cat stretch
- Standing pec stretch
- Lat stretch
- Shoulder stretch
- Neck stretch
- Bicep stretch
- Tricep stretch

STRENGTH TRAINING WORKOUT: 3 TIMES A WEEK

❏ ❏ ❏ Ballet squats .... 4 sets of 15 to 20 reps
❏ ❏ ❏ Calf raises .... 4 sets of 15 to 20 reps
❏ ❏ ❏ Basic crunches .... 4 supersets of 30 to 50 reps
❏ ❏ ❏ Advanced crunches .... 4 supersets of 30 to 50 reps
❏ ❏ ❏ Reverse crunches .... 4 supersets of 30 to 50 reps
❏ ❏ ❏ Dumbell presses .... 4 sets of 8 to 10 reps
❏ ❏ ❏ Pull-ups .... 4 sets of 8 to 10 reps
❏ ❏ ❏ Reverse-grip pulldowns .... 4 sets of 8 to 10 reps
❏ ❏ ❏ Barbell clean presses .... 4 sets of 10 to 12 reps
❏ ❏ ❏ Bent-over rear delt raises .... 4 sets of 10 to 12 reps
❏ ❏ ❏ Standing barbell curls .... 4 sets of 10 to 12 reps
❏ ❏ ❏ Cable bicep curls .... 4 sets of 10 to 12 reps
❏ ❏ ❏ Bench dips .... 4 sets of 10 to 12 reps
❏ ❏ ❏ Cable tricep extensions .... 4 sets of 10 to 12 reps
❏ ❏ ❏ Forearm extension .... 4 sets of 10 reps
❏ ❏ ❏ Forearm flexion .... 4 sets of 10 reps
❏ ❏ ❏ Forearm rotation .... 4 sets of 10 reps

117

CARDIO TRAINING WORKOUT: 30 MINUTES, 3 TIMES A WEEK

Type of cardio activity: _____

Interval training? ❏ Yes   ❏ No

STRETCHES: INCORPORATE INTO EACH DAY'S WORKOUT

• Quad stretch
• Glute stretches
• Inner thigh stretch
• Hamstring stretch
• Calf stretch
• Knee hug
• Back extensions
• Cat stretch
• Standing pec stretch
• Lat stretch
• Shoulder stretch
• Neck stretch
• Bicep stretch
• Tricep stretch

STRENGTH TRAINING WORKOUT: 3 TIMES A WEEK

☐ ☐ ☐ Flexed deadlifts .... 4 sets of 15 to 20 reps
☐ ☐ ☐ Calf raises .... 4 sets of 15 to 20 reps
☐ ☐ ☐ Basic crunches .... 4 supersets of 30 to 50 reps
☐ ☐ ☐ Advanced crunches .... 4 supersets of 30 to 50 reps
☐ ☐ ☐ Reverse crunches .... 4 supersets of 30 to 50 reps
☐ ☐ ☐ Bench push-ups .... 4 sets of 8 to 10 reps
☐ ☐ ☐ Single-arm dumbbell rows .... 4 sets of 8 to 10 reps
☐ ☐ ☐ Straight-arm lat pulldowns .... 4 sets of 8 to 10 reps
☐ ☐ ☐ Seated dumbbell presses .... 4 sets of 10 to 12 reps
☐ ☐ ☐ Dumbbell lateral raises .... 4 sets of 10 to 12 reps
☐ ☐ ☐ Standing barbell curls .... 4 sets of 10 to 12 reps
☐ ☐ ☐ Hammer curls .... 4 sets of 10 to 12 reps
☐ ☐ ☐ Overhead dumbbell extensions .... 4 sets of 10 to 12 reps
☐ ☐ ☐ Cable tricep extensions .... 4 sets of 10 to 12 reps
☐ ☐ ☐ Forearm extension .... 4 sets of 10 reps
☐ ☐ ☐ Forearm flexion .... 4 sets of 10 reps
☐ ☐ ☐ Forearm rotation .... 4 sets of 10 reps

118

CARDIO TRAINING WORKOUT: 30 MINUTES, 3 TIMES A WEEK

Type of cardio activity: _____

Interval training? ☐ Yes ☐ No

STRETCHES: INCORPORATE INTO EACH DAY'S WORKOUT

- Quad stretch
- Glute stretches
- Inner thigh stretch
- Hamstring stretch
- Calf stretch
- Knee hug
- Back extensions
- Cat stretch
- Standing pec stretch
- Lat stretch
- Shoulder stretch
- Neck stretch
- Bicep stretch
- Tricep stretch

STRENGTH TRAINING WORKOUT: 3 TIMES A WEEK

- ☐ ☐ ☐ One-leg leg presses .... 4 sets of 15 to 20 reps
- ☐ ☐ ☐ Calf raises .... 4 sets of 15 to 20 reps
- ☐ ☐ ☐ Basic crunches .... 4 supersets of 30 to 50 reps
- ☐ ☐ ☐ Advanced crunches .... 4 supersets of 30 to 50 reps
- ☐ ☐ ☐ Reverse crunches .... 4 supersets of 30 to 50 reps
- ☐ ☐ ☐ Standing cable flyes .... 2 sets of 8 to 10 reps
- ☐ ☐ ☐ Push-ups .... 2 sets of 8 to 10 reps
- ☐ ☐ ☐ Reverse-grip pulldowns .... 1 set of 8 to 10 reps
- ☐ ☐ ☐ Straight-arm lat pulldowns .... 1 set of 8 to 10 reps
- ☐ ☐ ☐ Pull-ups .... 1 set of 8 to 10 reps
- ☐ ☐ ☐ Single-arm dumbell rows .... 1 set of 8 to 10 reps
- ☐ ☐ ☐ Seated dumbbell presses .... 1 sets of 10 to 12 reps
- ☐ ☐ ☐ Bent-over rear delt raises .... 1 sets of 10 to 12 reps
- ☐ ☐ ☐ Dumbell lateral raises .... 1 set of 10 to 12 reps
- ☐ ☐ ☐ Barbell clean presses .... 1 set of 10 to 12 reps
- ☐ ☐ ☐ Cable bicep curls .... 1 set of 10 to 12 reps
- ☐ ☐ ☐ Hammer curls .... 1 set of 10 to 12 reps
- ☐ ☐ ☐ Standing barbell curls .... 1 set of 10 to 12 reps
- ☐ ☐ ☐ Alternating dumbbell curls .... 1 set of 10 to 12 reps
- ☐ ☐ ☐ Overhead dumbbell extensions .... 1 set of 10 to 12 reps
- ☐ ☐ ☐ Bench dips .... 1 set of 10 to 12 reps
- ☐ ☐ ☐ Dumbbell kickbacks .... 1 set of 10 to 12 reps
- ☐ ☐ ☐ Cable tricep extensions .... 1 set of 10 to 12 reps
- ☐ ☐ ☐ Forearm extension .... 3 sets of 12 to 15 reps
- ☐ ☐ ☐ Forearm flexion .... 3 sets of 12 to 15 reps
- ☐ ☐ ☐ Forearm rotation .... 3 sets of 12 to 15 reps

CARDIO TRAINING WORKOUT: 30 MINUTES, 3 TIMES A WEEK

Type of cardio activity: _____

Interval training? ☐ Yes ☐ No

STRETCHES: INCORPORATE INTO EACH DAY'S WORKOUT

- Quad stretch
- Glute stretches
- Inner thigh stretch
- Hamstring stretch
- Calf stretch
- Knee hug
- Back extensions

- Cat stretch
- Standing pec stretch
- Lat stretch
- Shoulder stretch
- Neck stretch
- Bicep stretch
- Tricep stretch

STRENGTH TRAINING WORKOUT: 3 TIMES A WEEK

❏ ❏ ❏ One-leg leg presses .... 1 set of 15 to 20 reps
❏ ❏ ❏ Ballet squats .... 1 set of 15 to 20 reps
❏ ❏ ❏ Flexed deadlifts .... 1 set of 15 to 20 reps
❏ ❏ ❏ One-legged squats .... 1 set of 15 to 20 reps
❏ ❏ ❏ Calf raises .... 4 sets of 15 to 20 reps
❏ ❏ ❏ Basic crunches .... 4 supersets of 30 to 50 reps
❏ ❏ ❏ Advanced crunches .... 4 supersets of 30 to 50 reps
❏ ❏ ❏ Reverse crunches .... 4 supersets of 30 to 50 reps
❏ ❏ ❏ Standing cable flyes .... 1 set of 8 to 10 reps
❏ ❏ ❏ Push-ups .... 1 set of 8 to 10 reps
❏ ❏ ❏ Incline bench presses .... 1 set of 8 to 10 reps
❏ ❏ ❏ Dumbbell presses .... 1 set of 8 to 10 reps
❏ ❏ ❏ Reverse-grip pulldowns .... 2 sets of 8 to 10 reps
❏ ❏ ❏ Straight-arm lat pulldowns .... 2 sets of 8 to 10 reps
❏ ❏ ❏ Pull-ups .... 2 sets of 8 to 10 reps
❏ ❏ ❏ Single-arm dumbbell rows .... 2 sets of 8 to 10 reps
❏ ❏ ❏ Seated dumbbell presses .... 2 sets of 10 to 12 reps
❏ ❏ ❏ Bent-over rear delt raises .... 2 sets of 10 to 12 reps
❏ ❏ ❏ Barbell clean presses .... 2 sets of 10 to 12 reps
❏ ❏ ❏ Dumbbell lateral raises .... 2 sets of 10 to 12 reps
❏ ❏ ❏ Cable bicep curls .... 2 sets of 10 to 12 reps
❏ ❏ ❏ Hammer curls .... 2 sets of 10 to 12 reps
❏ ❏ ❏ Standing barbell curls .... 2 sets of 10 to 12 reps
❏ ❏ ❏ Alternating dumbbell curls .... 2 sets of 10 to 12 reps
❏ ❏ ❏ Overhead dumbbell extensions .... 2 sets of 10 to 12 reps
❏ ❏ ❏ Bench dips .... 2 sets of 10 to 12 reps
❏ ❏ ❏ Cable tricep extensions .... 2 sets of 10 to 12 reps
❏ ❏ ❏ Dumbbell kickbacks .... 2 sets of 10 to 12 reps
❏ ❏ ❏ Forearm extension .... 3 sets of 12 to 15 reps
❏ ❏ ❏ Forearm flexion .... 3 sets of 12 to 15 reps
❏ ❏ ❏ Forearm rotation .... 3 sets of 12 to 15 reps

CARDIO TRAINING WORKOUT: 30 MINUTES, 3 TIMES A WEEK

Type of cardio activity: _____

Interval training? ❏ Yes ❏ No

STRETCHES: INCORPORATE INTO EACH DAY'S WORKOUT

- Quad stretch
- Glute stretches
- Inner thigh stretch
- Hamstring stretch
- Calf stretch
- Knee hug

- Back extensions
- Cat stretch
- Standing pec stretch
- Lat stretch
- Shoulder stretch

- Neck stretch
- Bicep stretch
- Tricep stretch

ABOUT
THE AUTHOR

BRAD HAMLER is an Atlanta-based fitness professional with more than 18 years' experience in the field, 15 of which were spent in New York City. He has been a personal training manager for Crunch Fitness; teaches classes such as Ultimate Conditioning, Abdominals Core Training, and Cardio-Conditioning; and has run his own company, Hamler Fitness Team, an in-house personal training business. He lectures and regularly holds seminars on golf and fitness as well as other fitness topics.

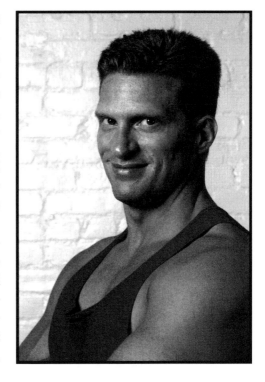

Brad has recently appeared on ABC-Channel 7, in New York, demonstrating his "No Gimmicks Workout," and on NBC Weekend Today, FOX Cable Morning, the MSG Channel, and "Daybreak with Beau Bock" in Atlanta. Brad also designed the workout in the CRUNCH Fitness Guide, *Beginner's Luck*, published by Hatherleigh Press in 1999.

Brad is originally from Ohio, where he began his career in fitness. He was a nationally ranked Natural Competitive Bodybuilder, and he has appeared in various fitness and bodybuilding publications. In addition to a B.A. in Business Administration from Findlay University, Brad has earned the following professional credentials: Master Trainer from the National Academy of Sports Medicine (NASM), Certified Personal Trainer (ACE), and Post-Rehab Conditioning Specialist (AAHFP).

NOTES

NOTES

NOTES